101 Tips

for Diabetes
Self-Management
Education

Martha Mitchell Funnell, MS, RN, CDE
Robert M. Anderson, EdD
Nugget Burkhart, RN, MA, CPNP, CDE
Mary Lou Gillard, MS, RN, CDE
Robin Nwankwo, MPH, RD, CDE

American Diabetes Association.
Cure • Care • Commitment℠

Director, Book Publishing, John Fedor; *Associate Director, Professional Books,* Christine B. Welch; *Editor,* Joyce Raynor; *Production Manager,* Peggy M. Rote; *Composition,* Circle Graphics, Inc.; *Cover Design,* Koncept Advertising and Design; *Printer,* Port City Press

Printed in the United States of America
1 3 5 7 9 10 8 6 4 2

The suggestions and information contained in this publication are generally consistent with the *Clinical Practice Recommendations* and other policies of the American Diabetes Association, but they do not represent the policy or position of the Association or any of its boards or committees. Reasonable steps have been taken to ensure the accuracy of the information presented. However, the American Diabetes Association cannot ensure the safety or efficacy of any product or service described in this publication. Individuals are advised to consult a physician or other appropriate health care professional before undertaking any diet or exercise program or taking any medication referred to in this publication. Professionals must use and apply their own professional judgment, experience, and training and should not rely solely on the information contained in this publication before prescribing any diet, exercise, or medication. The American Diabetes Association—its officers, directors, employees, volunteers, and members—assumes no responsibility or liability for personal or other injury, loss, or damage that may result from the suggestions or information in this publication.

⊗ The paper in this publication meets the requirements of the ANSI Standard Z39.48-1992 (permanence of paper).

ADA titles may be purchased for business or promotional use or for special sales. To purchase this book in large quantities, or for custom editions of this book with your logo, contact Lee Romano Sequeira, Special Sales & Promotions, at the address below, or at LRomano@diabetes.org or call 703-299-2046.

American Diabetes Association
1701 North Beauregard Street
Alexandria, Virginia 22311

Library of Congress Cataloging-in-Publication Data

101 tips for diabetes self-management education / Martha Mitchell Funnell. . . [et al.].
    p. cm.
  ISBN 1-58040-137-6 (pbk. : alk. paper)
    1. Diabetes—Miscellanea. 2. Self-care, Health—Miscellanea. 3. Patient education—Miscellanea. I. Title: One hundred one tips for diabetes self-management education. II. Funnell, Martha Mitchell.

RC660.4 .A146 2002
616.4'62—dc21

2002027663

To diabetes educators everywhere
who are dedicated
to improving the lives
of their patients.

CONTENTS

Introduction vii

Diabetes Self-Management Education Program
  Development 1

Defining your Vision 11

Designing the Curriculum 17

Evaluating your Program 25

Choosing and Using your Advisory Committee 33

Marketing your Program 41

Educator Issues and Concerns 47

Assessing Educational Needs 53

Content-Specific Issues 57

Meeting Individual Needs 69

Cultural Competency 79

Meeting the Needs of Special Populations 85

Educational Materials 95

Facilitating Group Sessions 111

Enhancing Teaching Skills .125

Challenging Patients 139

INTRODUCTION

This book contains a series of tips for providing self-management education for people with diabetes. Tips are included for both individual and group teaching and across the patient's lifespan. The information in these tips reflects the philosophy, experiences, and practice of the diabetes educators at the University of Michigan Diabetes Research and Training Center. It is our hope that you will find these tips helpful in your practice.

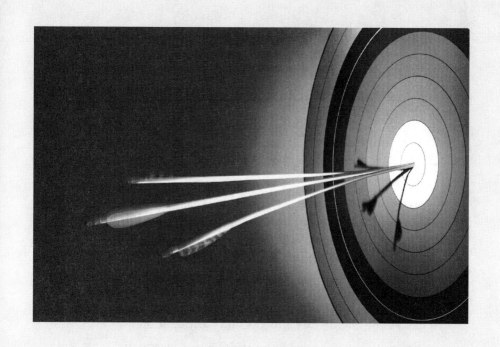

DIABETES

SELF-MANAGEMENT

EDUCATION PROGRAM

DEVELOPMENT

1

*W*hat are the National Standards for Diabetes Self-Management Education?

 Tip

The National Standards for Diabetes Self-Management Education are designed to promote quality diabetes education and are based on available scientific evidence. The Standards address the structure, process, and outcomes of diabetes education programs and offer guidelines related to assessment, content, instructor qualifications, evaluation, and organizational support. The ten content areas are

- describing the disease process and treatment options
- incorporating appropriate nutritional management
- incorporating appropriate physical activity
- utilizing medications
- monitoring blood glucose, monitoring urine ketones (when appropriate), and using the results to improve control
- preventing, detecting, and treating acute complications
- preventing (through risk reduction), detecting, and treating chronic complications
- goal-setting and problem-solving to promote health
- psychosocial adjustment
- preconception care, management of diabetes in pregnancy, and gestational diabetes management as needed

The Standards were first developed by organizations involved in diabetes care and education in 1985 and are reviewed every five years. The organizations, federal agencies, and programs that participated in the 2000 revision are: the American Diabetes Association (ADA), American Association of Diabetes Educators (AADE), American Dietetic Associa-

Tip *Continued*

tion, Veteran's Health Administration, Centers for Disease Control and Prevention, Indian Health Service, National Certification Board for Diabetes Educators, Juvenile Diabetes Research Foundation International, and Diabetes Research and Training Centers. Copies of the Standards are available from any of the participating organizations or online at www. diabetes.org/recognition/education.

2

How can I receive reimbursement from third-party payers for my diabetes self-management education (DSME) program?

 Tip

Payment for diabetes education is mandated in almost all 50 states. Most payers require educational programs to meet certain criteria and to be either nationally recognized or state certified. Education programs seeking Medicare reimbursement must be nationally recognized. The ADA offers a national recognition program for diabetes education programs. Its review criteria are based on the National Standards for Diabetes Self-Management Education.

Some states offer certification through their departments of public or community health or through their diabetes control programs. Some of these certification programs have their own standards, whereas others use the National Standards along with their own review criteria. A prescription that includes areas that need to be addressed is often required for reimbursement of diabetes self-management education (DSME).

The most efficient way to find out about requirements for reimbursement in your area is to contact other education programs, third-party payers, or the state insurance commissioner. If participants are denied insurance coverage even though you believe that diabetes education is a covered benefit, participants can contact their insurance company or the state insurance commissioner. Insurance commissioners are particularly appropriate contacts to respond to questions about reimbursement in states with mandated coverage.

3

Many of the participants in my DSME program are elderly. What do I need to do to be reimbursed by Medicare?

 Tip

The 1997 Balanced Budget Act included a provision for reimbursement for DSME and supplies. The Centers for Medicare and Medicaid Services (CMS) released their final ruling on the self-management education guidelines in December 2000. This ruling provides for a one-time benefit of ten hours of initial training and two hours per year of follow-up training from a nationally recognized outpatient program for DSME. CMS guidelines set aside one of the ten training hours for assessment in either a group or individual session. The remaining hours are to be used for group education. Two hours of follow-up per year may be provided in either a group or individual session. Participants with hearing problems or other special needs can receive the whole program in one-on-one sessions with a provider prescription. Medicare also provides reimbursement for three hours of Medical Nutrition Therapy (MNT) in addition to DSME.

To qualify for reimbursement for self-management education, Medicare beneficiaries must be newly diagnosed, not have received training at the time of their diagnosis, or be at significant risk for complications from diabetes. Patients must also have an A1C level of 8.5 or more on two consecutive measurements, three or more months apart.

4

What is a needs assessment and why is it important for a diabetes education program?

Tip

Effective program planning, implementation, and evaluation begins with a needs assessment. In order to be successful, diabetes education programs must understand and meet the needs of the the target population and the geographical area it intends to serve. The target population can include all people with diabetes or be limited to one or more groups of people with diabetes, such as only type 1 patients, the elderly, or children with diabetes. A program can also limit its scope to patients in a particular practice or managed care organization.

A needs assessment includes information about the demographic, cultural, social, and financial characteristics of the target population. You can also evaluate access and transportation issues for your service area and population. By carefully conducting a needs assessment of the community and the patients your program serves, you gain useful information for both planning and evaluating your education program.

5

I'm comfortable developing the educational content for our new DSME program, but I want to be sure that my program will be valued and used by the community. How can I conduct an effective needs assessment?

 Tip

A useful first step is to assess the character and needs of your community. You can use the following questions as a guide for collecting the information you will need to tailor your program to your target audience.

- Who is your target audience? From their point of view, what are the costs and benefits of attending your program? For example, would participants in your program have significant transportation costs or child care expenses or have to take time off from work to participate? If your program is offered close to meal times, will you provide refreshments?

- Are other diabetes education programs available for the same audience?

- What are the particular strengths and weaknesses of those programs in terms of availability, location, and cost?

- Does your program conflict with or support the other diabetes services provided at your institution?

- Have you assessed the diabetes education needs of patients who come to your setting for other services?

- Will you charge for your program? Is the cost reimbursed by most insurers in your area?

- Can you make special arrangements for patients who don't have insurance or adequate financial resources?

5

Tip *Continued*

■ Can you make your program a low-cost or free service by
identifying one or more sponsors who can offer full or partial
scholarships?

The answers to these questions will help you design a program that has
a high likelihood of meeting the needs of your target audience.

6

I've heard a number of the physicians, administrators, and third-party payers in my area say that DSME doesn't work. How can I respond to this statement?

 Tip

Generally, people who make this type of statement define education as giving patients information about diabetes self-management and then expecting patients to comply with their treatment plan. Giving patients information over a short period of time in hopes that they will make long-term behavior changes does not work.

However, most diabetes educators today have gone well beyond this outdated conceptualization of education. We have realized that education must address the entire person (i.e., psychosocial as well as clinical issues) and must focus on behavior, not just knowledge. Furthermore, patients need this behavioral and holistic type of education throughout the course of their illness. Expecting a patient to attend a self-management education program with no follow-up visits makes no more sense than if a patient visited a physician, got a prescription, and then never went back.

The sustained behavior change required for effective diabetes self-management requires ongoing support from a team of health care professionals and a periodic review and revision of the self-management plan to accommodate the changes in the patient's life or diabetes care. A number of review articles and meta-analyses in the literature demonstrate that this type of diabetes education is effective.

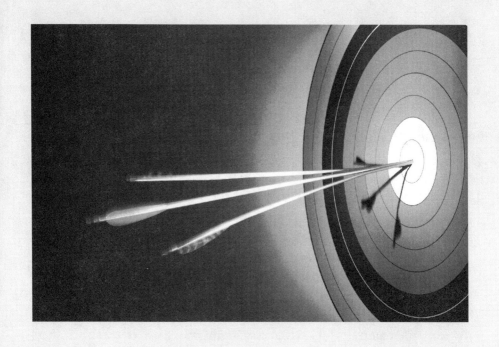

DEFINING

YOUR VISION

7

I've noticed that many organizations have mission statements or philosophies. Would developing a mission statement be a useful thing for our DSME program team to do?

 Tip

Yes. Writing a mission or philosophy statement helps your team to clarify and sharpen its understanding of your program's primary purpose. Once that fundamental purpose has been clearly established, deciding how to approach patients and provide education becomes much easier.

Collaborating on a mission statement also benefits the team by creating an opportunity to discuss and examine areas where team members may agree or disagree. Otherwise, disagreements about purpose and methods often do not emerge until the group has been working together for a significant amount of time. These differences can undermine the effectiveness of the program and can cause team members to give different messages to patients. Working on a mission statement can help members feel that they are part of a truly unified team.

Finally, developing a mission statement is part of meeting the National Standards for Diabetes Self-Management Education.

8

*H*ow can our DSME program team begin to define and articulate our mission statement?

 Tip

A mission statement is a reflection of the vision or philosophy of care. Our vision speaks to the larger goals and values that shape our work as health professionals. On a day-to-day basis, we may focus on short-term outcomes, such as helping patients develop the knowledge and skills required for effective diabetes self-management. However, helping patients become effective diabetes self-managers is a means to a larger end. That end is helping patients have longer, healthier, and more enjoyable lives.

When we begin to think about our purposes at that global level, we are beginning to articulate our vision. We once heard a physician remark, "What my patients want is fairly simple. They want to have a good life. My job is to help them have a good life." This simple and yet profound statement was the vision underlying the nuts and bolts of the diabetes care he provided to his patients.

A good way to begin defining your shared philosophy is to have each team member write a short vision statement, perhaps an answer to a question such as, "Why am I doing this work?" or "What is my overall purpose in being a diabetes educator?" The next step is to share and discuss the answers. Refining your personal vision helps you articulate your philosophy to others and provides a touchstone you can use to remain true to your beliefs. This process also lays the groundwork for developing the written vision statement that combines the key principles in each team members' answers into a coherent message.

9

My vision for diabetes education matches the empowerment philosophy. How can I be sure that my DSME program reflects this approach?

 Tip

In diabetes education, empowerment is defined as helping individuals discover and use their own innate ability to achieve mastery over their diabetes. There are two important areas to consider. The first is the way that we provide information. The second is the relationships we create with our patients.

Education for patient empowerment is designed to provide patients with the ability to make informed choices. The content is the same as in a traditional program, but diabetes management and treatment options are presented in the context of helping patients weigh costs and benefits and make the best decision for their lives. In addition, patients need to

- know how to make changes in their behavior and solve problems
- understand their role as a decision-maker and how their own goals, values, and feelings about diabetes influence their decisions
- know how to assume responsibility for their own care

Patients also need to acquire certain skills to assume this responsibility. They need to know how to maintain their own motivation, communicate effectively, and receive support from others in their environment. One of the patient's major activities is to develop goals for self-selected behavior change with his or her diabetes educator.

The empowerment philosophy envisions the relationship between patient and educator as a partnership. Our role is to serve as a collaborator and to support patients' efforts to be the primary decision-makers for

9

Tip *Continued*

their own care. The partnership is based on the understanding that knowing about diabetes is not the same as knowing what is best for that person.

The most fundamental and difficult shift needed to embrace this philosophy is that, as educators, we have to give up the traditional view that the purpose of education is for patients to become adherent or compliant with the treatment plan. Instead, we educate for informed, self-directed decision-making and problem-solving so patients can manage their diabetes as they choose.

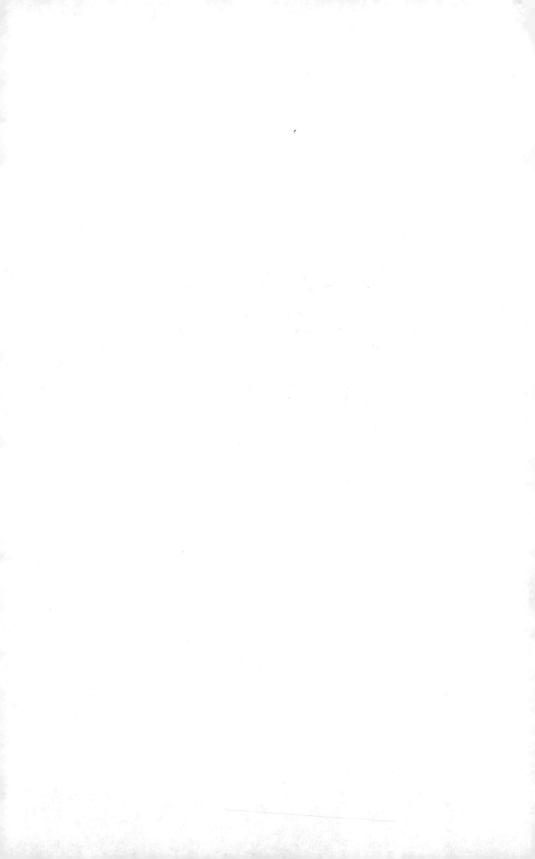

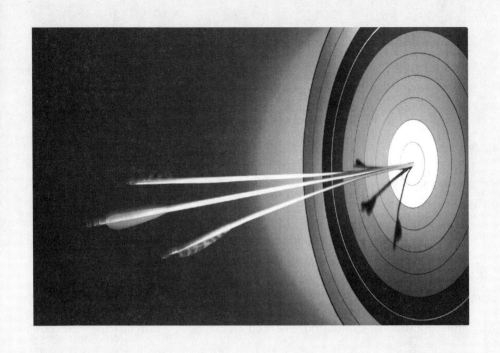

DESIGNING

THE CURRICULUM

10

I have been asked to develop a new diabetes self-management patient education program. Should I purchase an existing curriculum or develop my own?

 Tip

Y ou might want to do a little bit of both. There are excellent content outlines you can purchase that required hundreds of hours of work by a team of experts. Furthermore, they have been reviewed by experts and have proven helpful to diabetes educators in a variety of settings. These curricula include an overall goal and learning objective, a lesson plan, methodology, audiovisual instructional tools, participant handouts, and a method of evaluation. Such curricula can be purchased from ADA.

It doesn't make much sense to reinvent a curriculum that is already available and of high quality. However, to maximize the enthusiasm and effectiveness with which you teach the content, find a way to make it your own. For example, you, the other instructional team members and staff, and your program advisory committee can purchase content outlines suited to your patient population and then go through them in detail and add your own margin notes. You might want to include local or personal examples, or rephrase the material so it feels more like you. Personalizing a bought curriculum allows you to incorporate external material into your unique teaching approach and combine the best of both worlds.

11

I want to develop a problem-based education program in keeping with my vision of patient empowerment. What strategies can I use for this type of program?

 Tip

A problem-based DSME program relies on patient experiences. The problems and questions that the participants raise at each session are used to teach the necessary content areas. We use the following methods for providing a series of five two-hour class sessions.

We begin the first session by introducing ourselves, describing the program, and establishing ground rules. We let participants know that although we are experts in diabetes care, we are not experts on their lives. We also tell them the classes will be conducted differently than others they may have attended in that we rely on their expertise and questions. We then ask participants to introduce themselves and tell us what they would like to get from the program. We write their objectives on a flip chart and indicate if the content will be covered or if it is outside the scope of the program.

We then provide their own laboratory data to them using the form described in Tip 38 and ask if there are any questions. We close the session by providing goal-setting content and asking each person to identify a behavioral step or experiment he or she will try before the next session, one week later.

Session two begins with a discussion of the behavior-change experiments. We focus on what patients have learned from the week's efforts and their subsequent questions. We then ask what content areas they want to address, elicit further questions from the group, and respond with the appropriate content. This approach assures that information is always presented in response to the needs of class participants. All of the remaining sessions continue in this way. At the end of the last session, we review the list of participant objectives to be sure that all have been covered and

11

Tip *Continued*

ask each person, including the instructors, to identify one thing that the class has meant to them.

Two educators (a nurse and a dietitian in our case) lead the sessions of 10–15 participants, and both are experienced, flexible, and able to respond to questions introduced by patients in the order in which they are asked. Although the sessions are tiring for instructors because they have to pay very close attention and think on their feet, the sessions are also energizing because the participants' interest and enthusiasm remains high throughout the session.

12

*H*ow can I be sure that my problem-based
curriculum meets the National Standards so my
program can be reimbursed?

 Tip

everal factors help make a problem-based curriculum educationally
sound. For our program, we maintain a list of the content areas
required by the National Standards and check off topics discussed each
week. Because many topics are raised several times during the program,
instructors can reinforce and build on content that was presented earlier.
If there are areas that have not been addressed before the end of the program, we bring up the topic and ask if anyone has questions. Discussions
of psychosocial issues are included whenever initiated by patients and
facilitated by instructors within each content area. For example, when
discussing blood glucose monitoring, we ask how patients feel when they
have been working hard but still see a high number. We provide a
notebook of targeted handouts on all of the major content areas and
encourage participants to read the materials between classes and bring
them to each class session.

The key to providing essential content from the written curricula is to
respond to patient questions completely. This approach allows you to
address patient-identified problems and concerns and to provide an
educationally sound program.

13

My supervisor has asked me to write learning objectives for our DSME program. Do you have some advice about how to write effective learning objectives?

 Tip

Learning objectives describe the outcomes of the learning process. You can begin by asking yourself, "What should the participants in this group session be able to do at the end of the session that they could not do at the beginning?" The word "do" is important because effective objectives are always written in behavioral terms. In other words, observers should be able to agree that the participant has demonstrated the desired learning.

Objectives are divided into three domains: knowledge, skills, and attitudes. If your objective is in the knowledge domain, you will use terms such as "explain," "list," "state," or "describe." Because we can't directly observe what someone knows, it's important to describe a behavior that would demonstrate what participants know. For example: "At the end of this session, participants will be able to state their target blood glucose levels." Skills are a little easier because they are generally more amenable to observation. For example: "At the end of this session, participants will be able to demonstrate all the steps for using their blood glucose meter correctly."

The third domain is attitude and is especially difficult to measure. Attitudes are highly individual and may not be affected by information. Generally, attitudinal objectives are demonstrated through a changed score on a questionnaire or are verbalized by the patient. For example: "At the end of this session, participants will be able to verbalize the value of self-monitoring blood glucose for decision-making."

In summary, when writing objectives, ask yourself, "What would I have to see or hear to be convinced that the desired learning took place?"

14

I just finished writing objectives for our DSME program and ended up with 16 objectives for a one-hour group class. This seems like too many. How many objectives are reasonable?

 Tip

There is no hard and fast rule about the number of objectives per amount of instructional time. Generally, between two and six objectives per one hour of class time is a reasonable goal.

There are two probable explanations for developing 16 objectives for a one-hour class. One or both could apply to your situation. The first explanation is that the learning agenda is too ambitious for the period of time available. A way to judge length is by going through your objectives and writing down the estimated amount of time required for participants to acquire the knowledge or skill for each objective. Add up the total amount of time and see how well it matches the amount of time you had planned. Another possibility is that you are writing too many objectives. Some of these could perhaps be combined into a single objective. For example, if you have an objective for each of the steps involved in doing a blood glucose test, you probably have written too many. Instead, write one summary objective simply saying that participants will be able to demonstrate all of the steps necessary to monitor their blood glucose correctly.

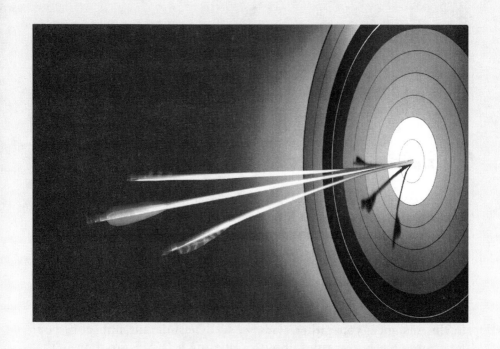

EVALUATING

YOUR PROGRAM

15

I need to evaluate my DSME program. Do you have any suggestions to help get me started?

 Tip

Remember that there are two distinct categories of evaluation. The first focuses on the educational process and is called formative evaluation. Formative evaluation involves gathering data from patients (e.g., using questionnaires) about what they considered the most and least helpful parts of the program. This information can help you improve the quality of the program and more closely match the needs of your patients.

The second evaluation category is summative or outcomes evaluation. In this instance, you gather evidence to determine the impact of your program. One of the rules about evaluating a DSME program is that measuring the most immediate impact of the program is usually easiest. For example, increased blood glucose monitoring can be linked more easily to the program than long-term outcomes, such as a reduction in complications.

Generally, the most immediate outcomes for DSME programs involve changes in knowledge, skills, and attitudes, followed by changes in self-management behavior, psychosocial adjustment, and care-seeking behavior. The AADE has developed an outcomes program called the National Diabetes Education Outcomes System (NDEOS). You can learn more about this tool by contacting AADE at (800) 338-3633 or www.aadenet.org.

16

*H*ow can I choose outcome measures for my DSME program?

 Tip

In addition to the formative evaluation and feedback that you gather from your patients, there are other dimensions you may want to examine as you evaluate the effectiveness of your program. Keep in mind that program evaluation is a continuing process and not a one-time event. The specific information gathered as part of your evaluation will help you make needed revisions to enhance the quality of your educational program.

Choose summative or outcome evaluation measures based on the goals of your program. An important question to ask yourself and to discuss with the other instructors or your advisory committee is, "Which outcomes can we expect to affect, considering our program and population?" (You really can't do it all.) This will help you determine which outcomes are most likely to demonstrate the effectiveness of your program. Choose outcomes that are consistent with your approach to diabetes education, curriculum, areas of emphasis, population, unique features, and your vision of your role as an educator.

Other dimensions to consider in evaluating your diabetes education program include

- the impact of your program on outcome measures collected pre- and postattendance
- the appropriateness or value of specific program objectives in relation to resources
- the effort (i.e., time, resources, and money) expended by specific program activities in meeting program objectives
- the performance of the program and the results of program activities

16

Tip *Continued*

- the effectiveness of specific program activities in addressing the goals of the program and in meeting the needs of the target population
- the efficiency of the program in terms of the goals achieved, needs met, or needs reduced in relation to the effort (i.e., time, resources, and money) expended

Finally, consider the process of implementing the program as well as the outcomes of the program. A process evaluation is an attempt to understand how or why a program met needs or achieved goals and is useful for improving the efficiency of the program.

*H*ow can I keep track of my participants' behavioral goal achievement in a way that is meaningful for them and useful for program evaluation purposes?

 Tip

Helping participants achieve the knowledge and skills they need to care for their diabetes and reach their goals is an important objective for most education programs. This means that many of the tools you use to assess the educational needs and evaluate the progress of individual participants can also help assess the effectiveness of your program. Examples include the use of knowledge tests, skills checklists, follow-up on behavior-change goals, and a goal attainment form to document changes in individual performance.

Using a goal record can help you to track each participant's self-selected goals and provides a system to rate the participant's level of attainment. The ratings will be more meaningful if both the participant and health professional complete them. The following scale can be used for each goal:

---

1 = Much less than expected level of attainment

2 = Less than expected

3 = Expected level of attainment

4 = More than expected

5 = Much more than expected level of attainment

In using this scale, both the educator and the patient need to understand that a rating of 3 is what is expected and means that the participant has met his or her goal. Instructors also need to understand that one of the purposes of recording goals is to provide patients with a way to reflect

17

Tip *Continued*

on their efforts, so the rating should be realistic and be determined by the participants.

Changing the habits of daily life is not an easy task. Diabetes self-management requires many difficult choices each and every day. We need to remember that people generally do the best they can—it's our job to provide information, facilitate their decision-making, and help them feel good about their efforts.

18

I need to do Continuous Quality Improvement (CQI) as part of meeting the DSME National Standards. What is CQI?

 Tip

Continuous Quality Improvement (CQI) is an ongoing process that helps ensure that the quality of the program is maintained. The steps for CQI are carried out in a cyclical manner so problems can be identified and resolved on a continuous basis. There are multiple variations of this process, but most generally, the following are included:

- identify the area for improvement
- collect and analyze data
- choose an approach
- develop the concepts and processes
- implement, evaluate, and improve the plan

Though seemingly cumbersome, this process is not unlike the steps that we teach patients to use for making continuous improvements in their self-management plan and setting goals for behavior change. CQI ensures that issues are identified and dealt with constantly so they don't become insurmountable problems or major crises.

CQI is a useful activity for meetings of the advisory committee or instructional team. Ask program participants, instructors, and members to identify problems or issues for each meeting and work through the process as a group. Incorporating due dates and responsible persons for each step will help ensure that tasks are carried out. Review the progress made and the results of CQI at each meeting. Remember, steps do not have to be successful to provide important information.

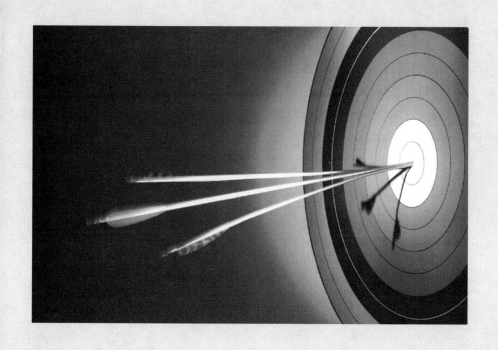

CHOOSING AND

USING YOUR

ADVISORY COMMITTEE

19

I know that I need an advisory committee to meet the National Standards for Diabetes Self-Management Education. What is the purpose of this group?

 Tip

An effective program advisory committee is made up of program stake-holders. Stakeholders have an investment in how well your program works. Your advisory committee *could* include

- one or more patients who can represent the target audience
- nurses
- dietitians
- a physician
- other relevant health care professionals, e.g., pharmacists, behaviorists
- an administrator

The advisory committee not only ensures that DSME standards are met, but also helps you review your curriculum and other materials, evaluate your program, conduct CQI, and market your program. When used effectively, your advisory committee can help you improve and maintain the quality of your program.

How can I choose professional members to be part of my DSME program advisory committee?

 Tip

The National Standards for Diabetes Self-Management Education recommend that the advisory committee be multidisciplinary, include at least a nurse and dietitian, and possibly include other professional team members such as a behaviorist, exercise physiologist, ophthalmologist, optometrist, pharmacist, physician, or podiatrist. Although you may not be able to include every professional group, it is helpful to include as many different professions as possible. One option is to include professions that represent areas where you feel least qualified to provide content that is important for your program. Also try to include stakeholders who have an interest in diabetes and in seeing your program succeed.

Choosing particular people to represent a discipline is a bit trickier. There are several considerations when choosing participants.

- Are they actively involved and identified with diabetes?
- Are they supportive of diabetes education in general and your program in particular? On the other hand, is it worth including a person who is difficult to work with or not supportive if he or she brings needed clout or other resources?
- Do they contribute to group discussions and work well with others in a committee situation?
- Do they honor commitments?
- Is their vision of diabetes care and education similar to yours?

Although not all professionals and disciplines that you might like to include are willing to serve on a committee, they might be willing to serve as a reviewer, a consultant on specific content areas or concerns, or a liaison to their colleagues.

21

I would like to include a consumer from the community on my program advisory committee, but on my previous committees, this person did not participate in discussions. Is there anything I can do to help this person feel more involved?

Tip

Think about it from the consumer's point of view. Most of the professionals on the committee interact on a professional basis. You have an established relationship and respect for each other's expertise. The consumer is in many ways a stranger and an outsider. Even though this person may receive care from committee members, he or she probably does not know you in the same way that you know each other.

If you are the advisory committee chair, it is up to you to be sure that each member is made to feel welcomed and valued. Acknowledging the expertise of the consumer and asking for advice with statements such as, "Based on your experiences with diabetes (or as a community leader), what do you think about . . . ?" can help. You might consider asking consumer members to make a short presentation to the group about their experiences or professional role so that they are viewed as an important contributor to the discussion. Even if you are not the chair of the committee, you still have a role in helping the consumer members feel valued by listening to what they have to say, not interrupting, and offering differing opinions in a way that does not personally attack or denigrate the other person.

With some support, consumers bring a new dimension to the patient education process and can bring out the best in other committee members.

22

*H*ow can I help the physicians in my area become more involved in and supportive of my DSME program?

 Tip

Many physicians view education as the role of nurses, dietitians, and other health care professionals. They may not recognize that they have a very important role to play.

One way to help physicians become involved in your education program is to meet with the key physicians who see many patients with diabetes. Ask those physicians what is important for them in the educational process and how they would like to be kept informed of their patients' progress in your program. Provide brochures for their office staff or waiting room. Let them know that patient education can save them time during office visits and can help their patients achieve behavioral goals and become more active participants in their care. Another way is to invite one or more key physicians to be on your advisory committee. This physician (or physicians) then becomes a stakeholder in the program and can help promote it to his or her colleagues.

Another strategy is to invite a physician that you respect to teach one session or attend a class in order to give you feedback on your content and teaching style. This not only provides valuable information for you, but also gives the physician the firsthand experience of seeing how patients respond to education.

Another way to help physicians become more involved in your program is to let them know how important they are in the referral process. While physicians rarely have time to provide education, telling patients how strongly they feel about the importance of education and encouraging patients to take advantage of the referral carries a great deal of weight and makes patients much more likely to attend.

Choosing and Using your Advisory Committee

23

I am the chairperson for our DSME program
advisory meetings. Do you have any tips for
running a successful meeting?

 Tip

One way to begin thinking about what makes a good meeting is to
focus on the two major needs that have to be met in almost all meetings. The first and most obvious needs are tasks, i.e., accomplishing the
work identified on the meeting agenda. The second need may be less
obvious—positive working relationships among those attending the meeting. For example, a committee that meets regularly might want to spend
the first few minutes catching up with each other about what is going on
in their lives or their work. Although this may seem to be "off task," it
isn't. For a group to function smoothly, people must feel connected to the
other members of the group.

One of the responsibilities of a group leader is to judge how much time
to spend on relationship issues and how much to spend on task issues.
This ratio can vary for a number of reasons, including how long the
group has been functioning together and how often members interact
with each other outside the meeting. Groups that have worked together
for a long time usually need to devote less time to nurture relationships
than groups with members who don't know each other well.

Another way to improve meeting efficacy is to avoid having group members give oral reports simply to bring other members up to date. Instead,
ask each group member to submit any reports they have in writing or by
e-mail so they can be distributed and read before or brought to the meeting. Rather than asking for a summary of the report, invite questions from
the other members. The time that people are together is precious and can
be better used if the group focuses on important decisions and problems.

Another strategy is to have a written agenda with times next to each
item, e.g., Opening Remarks, 8:00 a.m., Approve Minutes, 8:10 a.m.,
Discuss Budget, 8:15 a.m., etc. This will allow you to quickly determine
whether you are behind, ahead, or on schedule during the meeting. These
simple suggestions can improve the efficiency and harmony of meetings.

*A*ttendance at advisory committee meetings for
my DSME program is really poor. What can I do
to encourage members to attend?

 Tip

L ow attendance at meetings indicates a lack of interest. Try to determine if the loss of interest is in the program or in the meeting itself.

When people agree to participate on your committee, they often do so
because they genuinely want to contribute to the program and to feel as
though that contribution is valued. Ask yourself if members of the committee have had the opportunity to contribute in a meaningful way. Were
the expectations clear when they agreed to be a member? Are the meetings conducted so members leave feeling that they have been active
participants? Do you listen more than you talk? Using meeting time to
just give reports or review written reports feels like a waste of time and
probably works negatively. Also, start and end on time and cover the
agenda efficiently while allowing adequate time for discussion.

Several activities that both contribute to the program and increase
involvement and attendance are as follows:

- Ask members to review particular content areas and handout
  materials on an annual basis and then have an open discussion
  of the curriculum.
- Feature particular members at each meeting by asking them to
  provide information about their particular area of interest.
- Invite a patient to attend and provide information to the group
  about his or her experiences with the program.
- Review the evaluation and outcomes data and discuss their
  implications.
- Hold a group brainstorming session about solutions for a particular problem or issue.

If you feel that the meetings are already conducted in a way that
promotes participation, talk with individual members about ways to
increase participation and attendance.

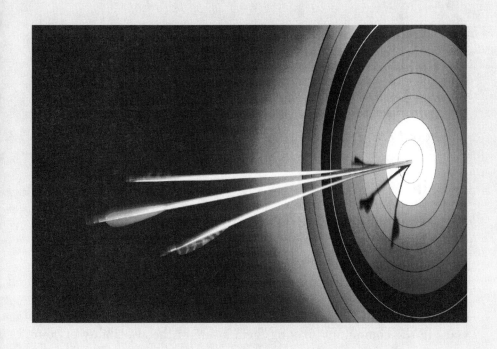

MARKETING

YOUR PROGRAM

25

I have developed a new DSME program that I think could provide real benefits to people in my community. Do you have any suggestions about how I can begin to advertise my program?

 Tip

If you have not already done so, this would be a great time to put together an advisory committee. The advisory committee can help you market your program to the target audience in a variety of ways.

You can ask each member to market your program within his or her particular constituency. For example, if you have a physician on your advisory committee, ask him or her to send a letter to the other physicians in the community making them aware of the availability of your program. Offering to write a first draft of the letter and handle all of the work and expense of mailing will increase the likelihood that a busy physician will provide this kind of support. Nurses, dietitians, pharmacists, and providers and administrators can make sure the word gets out within their own professional groups as well as refer patients to your program.

Your patient representatives can tell you how they typically learn about offerings and events in the community. Do they listen to particular radio stations? Are there free weekly newspapers that provide such information? Does your hospital have a marketing department that could help you access a radio or television commentator or a newspaper columnist friendly to your institution and interested in health stories? Does your local newspaper have a health reporter who might do a story about your new program? If your patient representative has already completed the program, he or she may be willing to be interviewed for a newspaper or television story.

Tip *Continued*

Including key community leaders on your committee can help direct marketing efforts to your target audience. Can they identify community events, such as health fairs, where you can provide brochures about your program? Are they part of community groups that might invite you to give a talk about diabetes and allow you to market your program?

Finally, over time you will have an increasing number of satisfied customers who can spread the word about your DSME program.

26

I do not seem to be getting much response from flyers about my program. Do you have any tips for making flyers more effective?

Tip

Think about what you look for when you are quickly scanning a flyer or advertisement. Most readers pay attention to how the advertised product or event relates to them. So, the first part of the flyer needs to highlight benefits to the readers or they may not read the rest of the flyer.

Bold this first part of your message and use a larger font for better impact. An example is: **Free Screening**! For maximum impact, place the next bolded message lower on the flyer, describing where and when the event will be held and spelling out the day and time. Follow this with the contact information. Boxing the contact information (including a phone number) will set it off as important reference information and will help the reader find it quickly.

In the next section, further describe what the reader will receive at the event (e.g., cholesterol screening, blood pressure measurements, workshops on diabetes care). Short phrases such as, "call for an appointment" help keep the flyer uncluttered and easy to read.

Always include the sponsoring organization, usually at the bottom of the page so as not to draw attention away from the key information.

27

I have a limited budget. Do you think giving away items that advertise my DSME program is a good use of my program dollars?

 Tip

For many diabetes educators, the answer will be yes. In today's health care climate, it may not be enough to offer a good program. To survive and thrive, you may need to market your program and services throughout your community.

When selecting an advertising tool, think about your program's core messages and choose items that fit your message. One example is a mirror with the message "Can you see yourself in control?" Choosing magnifying glasses for eye programs or pill boxes for "ask the pharmacist" events reinforces the theme of the event. Ballpoint pens are always welcomed at community fairs. Always include the name and telephone number of your program, using at least two lines.

We have found that business card magnets with simple messages, such as "Take care of you by taking care of your diabetes," are both useful and inexpensive. The cost of having a graphic artist design a program logo may be worth the one-time expense because incentives can be reordered using the same graphic multiple times.

There are many companies in the United States that specialize in the sale of such items, usually referred to as "premiums." To find premiums, check out the links at www.adspecialites.com.

28

*M*edia outlets in my community have been helpful in promoting our new DSME program, but I am worried they will forget about us. How can I keep the relationships going?

 Tip

One strategy to help maintain this network for future promotional events is to send a thank-you letter to the media personnel and to your organization's marketing department letting them know that their efforts were successful. Success can be measured by the number of people who indicated hearing about the program through the radio, television, or newspaper ads or stories. Including information regarding the number of calls you received on the day or week that the ad ran also gives positive feedback to the media and helps maintain your relationship with them.

You can also send letters to the managers of the television and radio station emphasizing your positive experience. Include the number of respondents as a result of the ad or story and the name of the reporter. When you contact them to market a new event, you can refer to your past successful venture.

Regularly provide your media contacts with public service announcements or, when your budget allows, paid advertisements. This emphasizes your allegiance and supports your relationship with them.

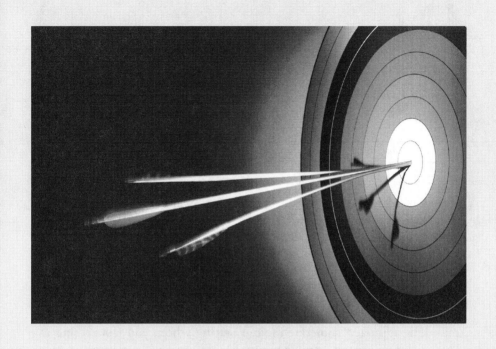

EDUCATOR

ISSUES

AND CONCERNS

29

I was just hired to work in a DSME program, and I am feeling overwhelmed! Where do I start?

 Tip

Starting out as a diabetes educator can feel overwhelming. Don't expect to learn everything overnight.

There are several ways that you can begin to build your knowledge base and create your vision as an educator. The other health professionals that you work with can be excellent resources. By watching other educators, physicians, nurses, and psychologists, you will learn about diabetes and about different styles of working with patients and families. You might approach someone in your setting whom you respect and ask if he or she will serve as your mentor. Working with a mentor or coach is extremely valuable. He or she can give you feedback and help you network within the professional diabetes care community.

Joining organizations for diabetes professionals such as ADA (www.diabetes.org), AADE (www.aadenet.org), your own professional association, and local branches of these organizations will provide you with information about conferences, professional publications, and materials for patients. They will also help you get in touch with other diabetes professionals working throughout your state and across the country.

How can I advance professionally as a diabetes educator and continue to learn about diabetes care and education?

 Tip

Attending professional meetings that focus on diabetes education and management will increase your knowledge. The ADA, AADE, American Dietetic Association, and other professional associations offer educational programs throughout the year that address the needs of educators at different levels of expertise, from basic to advanced.

Books published by ADA for professionals and patients are excellent resources, as is the *Core Curriculum for Diabetes Education*, published by AADE. Many professions offer standards of professional practice that are useful guides for professional growth.

You can consider becoming a Certified Diabetes Educator (CDE). Studying for the CDE examination will also help you focus your learning. You will need to work in diabetes education and management for at least two years before you are eligible to take the exam. Working toward this goal will give you a framework for your learning. For more information, contact the National Certification Board for Diabetes Educators (NCBDE) at (847) 228-9795 or at www.ncbde.org.

There is also a multidisciplinary advanced credential for nurses, dietitians, and pharmacists. This credential and the required examination are sponsored by the American Nurses Credentialing Center (ANCC) and AADE in collaboration with the ADA, the American Dietetic Association's Diabetes Care and Education Practice Group, the American Pharmaceutical Association, and NCBDE. For more information, contact ANCC at (800) 284-2378 or at www.nursecredentialing.org.

31

As an educator, I sometimes feel that no one values what I do. How can I show others in my organization that what I do has value?

 Tip

First, you need to value what you do! It helps to have a strong sense of purpose and receive gratification from creating relationships with patients and from doing your job well. You won't always get a pat on the back from your colleagues. You also need to know your vision and your goals and keep them in your sight at all times. Creating a vision and performance plan for yourself and reviewing it periodically helps you evaluate your progress.

Don't wait for others to discover the contribution that you make; bring your work to their attention. Write an article for the hospital newsletter about diabetes and your program. Submit an annual report to your administrator and program director highlighting accomplishments that demonstrate the program's value to patients and to your organization. Spread good will about the program by involving yourself in community activities related to diabetes.

32

Where can I get the support that I need to do my work?

 Tip

Networking with other educators who are dealing with similar issues and problems can be very supportive. Brainstorming with these colleagues can save you time and may prevent you from reinventing the wheel. Seasoned educators can offer helpful hints, resources, and support.

Networking also gives you contacts for when you need help with patient referrals or other issues. Getting involved with your area ADA, AADE, or your professional association will put you in touch with others involved in diabetes care.

33

I sometimes feel "burned out" as a diabetes educator. I want to give my patients and families the best care and education that I can. What can I do?

 Tip

Providing diabetes care and education takes lots of energy and enthusiasm. Take good care of yourself! If you are drained all the time, then you won't have anything to offer your patients.

Create a care plan for yourself. First, assess your current situation and try to pinpoint the issues. Be sure that you are looking at the big picture.

- Are you getting enough sleep?
- Are you eating well?
- Do you get enough exercise?
- Is there enough fun and enjoyment in your life?
- Are you taking the time to nurture your spiritual self?
- Are you working too many hours?
- What are the needs at work that are competing for your time?
- What are the needs at home that are competing for your time?
- Is your life in balance?
- Do you need to make any changes?

  - List those things over which you have control.
  - Prioritize your list to address the most problematic issue first.
  - Focus on steps you can take to solve your priority problem.
  - Make a commitment to take one step today.

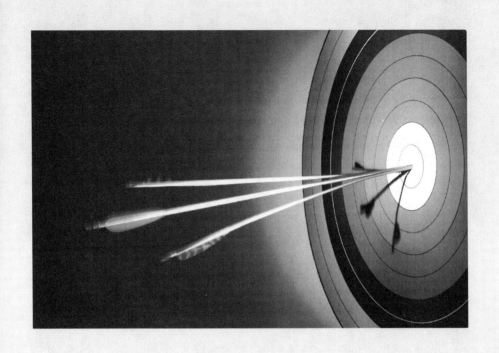

ASSESSING

EDUCATIONAL

NEEDS

34

I teach large classes and don't always have the opportunity to review the individual assessments prior to class. Is there a brief assessment I can do in class that could help guide my teaching?

Tip

Try asking participants to say a few words about what they have heard or what they know about diabetes. Their answers will not only help you assess current knowledge and educational needs, but also will allow you to detect any myths or incorrect beliefs that need to be cleared up before beginning your instruction.

For example, imagine if someone in your group were to say, "My grandmother had diabetes and went blind. That's how I know that diabetes causes you to lose your eyesight." Until this person realizes that diabetes doesn't have to lead to blindness, he or she probably won't be able to assimilate other information about diabetes and its self-management.

Another way to do a brief assessment is to ask participants why they came or what they hope to learn from the program. Write down the responses on a flip chart. Let participants know if there are areas you will not cover. Refer back to this list at the end of the program to be sure that you have covered all of the needs and topics identified.

Sometimes when I ask participants why they are attending my program, they say, "My doctor sent me." I worry that these participants won't get anything from the classes. Do you have any suggestions for how I can best work with them?

 Tip

Try having a private discussion with these patients. First, ask why they think their doctor sent them to a DSME program. Then ask whether they disagree with the doctor's judgment. If they disagree with their doctor's referral, ask why. They may disagree because of a previous experience with DSME or a lack of knowledge about the seriousness of diabetes, the risk for complications, or the impact of diabetes self-management on outcomes.

If patients have had negative experiences with DSME in the past, ask why it didn't work for them. Point out the ways in which your program is similar and different from others they have attended. Tell them your vision of education and ask if they are comfortable with this vision. Keep in mind that this is not the time to sell your program, but to help the patient decide if attending is the best use of his or her time and resources.

Some patients harbor the mistaken belief that if their symptoms are mild, then the disease is mild. Use the patient's most recent A1C value to objectively discuss his or her risk for complications.

Some patients may indicate that they know what to do, but they just don't do it. Ask these patients what would help them make changes and then tell them how your program will or will not meet those needs. You can use this discussion to help patients understand that the decisions they make every day, many of them involving the routine conduct of their lives, will have more impact on their health and well-being than the decisions made by health care professionals. You can also point out that when patients have more information, they are more able to choose behaviors and make decisions that result in better outcomes.

36

I am always concerned when I encounter newly diagnosed patients in my DSME program. How can I find out how they are coping with their diagnosis?

 Tip

Ask them to tell you their story. Most of us appreciate being asked about ourselves by someone who is interested and willing to listen.

Ask patients questions that help them think about their experiences rather than just the technical aspects of diabetes. Such questions include the following:

- How were you diagnosed?
- How were you told you had diabetes?
- How did you feel when you found out?
- Was it a surprise, or did you expect it?
- What did you do on the way home from the doctor's office that day?
- Who did you tell?
- What was your family's reaction to the diagnosis?
- What have you done to cope with diabetes since your diagnosis?
- How well do you feel you are coping with diabetes? What would help you to feel more at peace about having diabetes?

You can use these questions to initiate a conversation during an individual interaction or as part of a class activity. You can read the questions aloud to the class and ask participants to jot down what comes to mind. Then have them pick a partner and each spend five minutes discussing their answers. By helping patients to express, explore, and reflect on their experiences with diabetes, this exercise can provide valuable insight and facilitate coping.

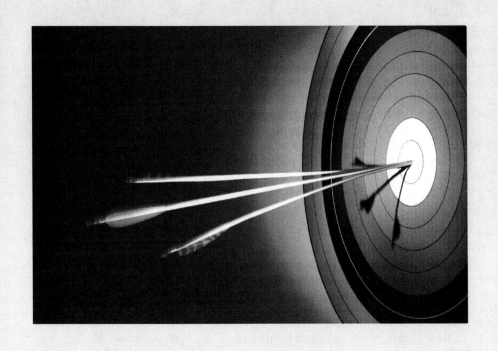

CONTENT-SPECIFIC

ISSUES

37

I struggle with how to present psychosocial content effectively. Can you offer some ideas?

 Tip

Many educators feel uncomfortable with psychosocial content and tend to put it at the end of their programs. Educators often hesitate to bring up the emotional difficulties of living with diabetes because we want our patients to think positively and focus on success. We also feel uncomfortable because we don't know how to respond or how to "fix" a patient's difficult feelings.

Diabetes doesn't have psychosocial problems—it is one. Almost every aspect of our patients' lives is affected. When patients think about diabetes, they think of it as a totality that includes psychosocial and physiological impacts.

An effective way to deal with the psychosocial aspects of diabetes is to integrate them throughout the entire curriculum. Almost every aspect of diabetes self-management has a psychosocial component, and patients are often anxious to talk about these issues. For example, content about hypoglycemia recognition, treatment, and prevention can be paired with a discussion of fear, embarrassment, or other emotional responses that participants have had as a result of this acute complication.

When faced with psychosocial issues, educators often respond with technical questions or information because we feel more confident in these areas. An example is a patient saying that he or she hates his or her diet and an educator responding by asking how many calories the patient has each day. Although the number of calories may indeed be a problem, a more appropriate response might be, "It sounds as if you have strong feelings about your meal plan. Can you tell me more about that?" Such a response allows the patient to feel safe and valued. It also gives the patient the opportunity to reflect on his or her feelings and explore how those feelings are influencing his or her behavior. Keep in mind that negative feelings can't be solved. Even though we like to help our patients feel better, ignoring psychosocial issues or offering information or advice in response to an expression of negative feelings is a disservice.

38

Many of my patients don't seem interested in learning about lab values and what they mean. How can I pique their interest?

 Tip

Most people are interested in learning about things that they believe have a direct impact on their lives. We find that using participants' own lab values is an effective way to teach this content. To facilitate discussion, we developed a form with three sections. The first section lists normal or ideal values for A1C, lipids, creatinine, microalbumin, and blood pressure and gives a brief explanation of each test. The second section contains each participant's most recent test values. You can fill in each patient's test score or, if you don't have that information, ask patients if they know their own test values. Encourage patients who don't know their test values to take the form to their next provider appointment to obtain the information. The third section of the form includes a place where patients can write down their own goals for each measurement.

Our form also includes a highlighted box that lists different behaviors that could help participants work toward a goal in each area. For example, the box under A1C says,

To help lower your blood sugar, you can

- eat fewer sweets
- eat smaller portions
- change how often you eat
- exercise more
- take medicine (pills or insulin)
- take a different medicine
- take a combination of medicines (pills and insulin)
- add or adjust insulin dose, timing, or number of shots per day

38

Tip *Continued*

Most people outside of the health care profession aren't interested in learning about lab values per se, but they are very interested in knowing their own lab values and what they mean. Providing individual values enlivens the discussion because the values are meaningful to each participant. Also, educators don't need to judge patients' test values as good or bad because the form lists normal or desired values for patients to make their own comparisons. In addition to teaching the meaning of lab values, this strategy often helps participants focus on areas or behaviors they might want to address when setting goals.

39

I tell my patients that A1C is a long-term measure of blood sugar that is an average of their blood sugar over the last two to three months. Many of them have difficulty understanding this concept. Do you have any suggestions?

 Tip

Patients need to understand what the A1C value means *clinically* and what it means *personally*. To help them understand the clinical relevance, compare their A1C result with the corresponding blood glucose level for their A1C number. There are a variety of ways to depict this graphically, for example, by using a thermometer or a stoplight. This helps the patients relate A1C numbers to their blood sugars and gives meaning to this lab value. Defining A1C as an average is not really accurate and may make A1C more complicated for patients to understand.

A more important part of the educational process is to teach patients what A1C means for them. Many patients do not understand that their A1C level gives them important information about their risk for diabetes complications. One way to convey this point is to show patients graphs from the Diabetes Control and Complications Trial (DCCT) comparing A1C levels to the incidence of complications. Help patients locate their A1C value on the graphs. In a class situation, you can show or draw this graph and have participants find where their A1C falls. Show patients that a 1% improvement in A1C has a significant impact on their risk for complications.

Once the participants understand the role of A1C and its implications on a personal level, you can ask patients where they would like to have their A1C level and what steps they will take to reach this goal.

40

What do I do when I try something with a patient and sometimes it works and sometimes it doesn't? For example, the patient gets different responses in his or her blood sugars when adjusting for exercise.

 Tip

Dealing with the unpredictability of diabetes is difficult for patients and the health care team. It is part of what makes diabetes so challenging. Patients seldom have the exact response from the same intervention on two separate occasions. Diabetes management is definitely not an exact science, but an art. Using trial and error to test new strategies is often the best way to make progress.

Patients who expect only positive and consistent results can become frustrated and give up. Let them know each person is different and that some things will work for them and others will not. They also need to know that their response will vary at different times. Encourage them to try a strategy and monitor to see if it works for them. This will both decrease their frustration and help them become more involved in their self-management.

Some of my patients are really nervous about giving themselves shots. How can I help them?

 Tip

For many nurses and other health professionals, giving injections is routine, almost automatic. But for patients who have just learned that they need to take insulin, giving themselves an injection is a *major* undertaking! They may envision a needle that is six inches long with the diameter of a pencil.

One approach is to have patients get the worst part out of the way before giving them a lot of information. They are often too anxious to listen or learn well. Start by giving patients an empty syringe and let them get the feel of it. Then, with the syringe still empty, have patients poke it into their own abdomen. This alleviates some of the anxiety concerning the manual dexterity needed to fill the syringe and the tension that mounts as they "load" the syringe knowing they must then "shoot" themselves. Even with the pen devices on the market today, getting to the "shooting" part first usually helps decrease the anxiety that blocks learning. Once they have actually poked themselves, they are better able to listen when you explain how to draw up or dial the dosage.

Some educators have invited a particularly fearful patient to inject the educator, or the educator has injected himself or herself. If you do this, be careful not to be too cavalier. Letting patients know that injections are not completely painless is more helpful then telling them that they don't hurt at all.

42

I feel embarrassed talking about sexual health with participants, especially in a group class. How can I feel more comfortable?

 Tip

Most of us were taught that sex is private or even dirty. Overcoming the messages that we learned as children is not easy. Cultural and other beliefs can also make talking about sex and sexual dysfunction difficult. Think about why you are uncomfortable and consider whether or not you first need to give yourself new messages about sex as a normal and healthy part of everyone's life.

There are things you can do to desensitize yourself so that you feel more comfortable. In front of a mirror or a colleague, practice your talk and use any words that are difficult to say or that make you giggle. Try talking about sexual issues with just one patient before you discuss the topic in a group. Talking with someone who is of a similar age and gender is usually easier. Gradually expand the number and variety of patients with whom you speak.

Most patients are grateful for information about sexual health and sexual functioning and will appreciate that you addressed this concern with them. Adopting a professional and matter-of-fact approach conveys that you are comfortable with the topic and helps patients feel at ease and free to ask questions.

43

I am a nurse and have not had a lot of exposure to nutrition. Now I have to do it all in my program. Is there an easy way to begin teaching about nutrition?

 Tip

Begin by asking the patient for his or her meal pattern for one day. Place each food item in the appropriate category on the food guide pyramid for a quick assessment of a patient's current diet. If three food categories have been included, then the meal has a balance of food groups. A 24-hour recall of foods eaten allows you to determine whether serving amounts approximate recommendations. Next, ask patients the following:

- How closely does this meal reflect your usual intake?
- What is different from day to day?
- How many meals are typically eaten on most days?
- What are your preferred foods—breads, fruits, vegetables, or meats?

You can now use the usual intake information to teach about portions, carbohydrate sources and amounts, types of fats, and how to adjust these foods for activity and medications.

44

My patients ask me, "What can I eat?" How can I respond?

 Tip

Try responding with another question such as, "What do you like to eat?" or "What do you want to eat?" Your questions will help refocus the discussion away from the more global world of nutrition and onto that particular patient's preferences. Once your patient identifies specific concerns about meal planning, you can provide the relevant information.

Questions also open the door to discussing other meal-planning issues. For example, you can ask patients about other aspects of meal planning such as who cooks, mealtime routines, limited cooking time or ability, and food shopping. Ask how they make food choices and how they evaluate the impact of those choices. This can provide useful information about how the meal plan is lived out and may highlight areas where the patient needs additional information.

My patients struggle with carbohydrate counting. Is there a way to teach carb counting that will make it easier for them?

 Tip

The first step is to help patients understand carbohydrates. Most of us do not think of our food as carbohydrates, proteins, or fats. The following is an activity we have used and found to be effective in both individual and group sessions. Use a food label as an example and an individual target for carbs per meal.

Start by writing down what the patient ate for his or her most recent meal. In a group class, ask one person to identify a meal or ask the group to identify favorite foods for a meal such as breakfast. Then, ask the patient(s) to identify the carbs at that meal. Record the amount of carbs next to the food. You can refer back to the food pyramid and exchange list to obtain the amount of carbs in each food. Add up the amount of carbs with the patient and compare with the target amount of carbs per meal. Ask the patient if he or she is surprised by the results. Then ask the patient to suggest modifications to the meal, such as smaller portions. We suggest blood glucose monitoring to determine if the amount of carbohydrate was too much or too little.

We find this activity is especially useful for what patients deem as a "bad" meal (e.g., meals where desserts, high-fat foods, or large portions were eaten). It helps patients to see the impact of portions and particular foods on carbohydrate intake. Food labels and food models can be used to reinforce these points.

This activity often provides a springboard to discuss fats and proteins and their effects on health and weight. Patients can then understand carbs as food and not just another word. A helpful book available from the ADA (http://store.diabetes.org) is *Practical Carbohydrate Counting: A How-to-Teach Guide for Health Professionals* by Hope S. Warshaw and Karen M. Bolderman, 2001.

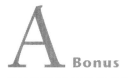

Bonus

I find that participants do not seem to be listening when I talk to them about complications. I think this is critical information. What can I do to make it more interesting?

 Tip

People with diabetes tell us that hearing and thinking about the complications of diabetes are the hardest parts of diabetes education. If you do not have diabetes, imagine having to hear about the potential for very serious and possibly fatal complications of an illness you have. The problem may not be a lack of interest, but rather anxiety and fear that causes the participants to tune out or avoid listening.

One approach is to start any discussion about complications with a good news/bad news introduction. The bad news is that complications can and do happen to people with diabetes, no matter how well they manage their blood sugar levels. The good news is that we know more about how to prevent complications, we have better treatment methods so blood sugar levels can stay closer to normal more easily, and we have better treatments for complications once they occur. Stress what participants can do to detect complications early when treatment is most effective. State the critical importance of blood glucose and blood pressure control for decreasing the risk of complications, but acknowledge that there are no guarantees.

Many participants have seen the devastating effects of diabetes on family and friends. Let them know that the disease is "not your grandmother's diabetes" anymore. Better treatments and research efforts offer hope that complications can be both prevented and treated.

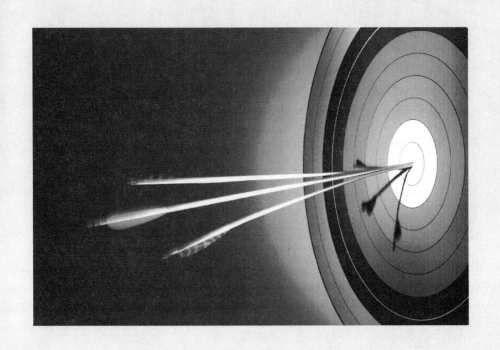

MEETING

INDIVIDUAL

NEEDS

46

Some of my patients believe in home remedies to treat diabetes and other problems. How can I assess their use of alternative therapies?

 Tip

Many patients take both alternative and conventional medicines. Because of the frequency with which patients use alternative medicines, it is appropriate to ask all patients, "Which vitamin, mineral, or other natural supplements do you take?" rather than asking *if* they use these products.

Determine if the patient has substituted an alternative practice or substance for prescribed medications. If so, you, the patient, and his or her physician need to discuss the implications of such a decision.

However, most patients add alternative health care practices to their existing self-management program. In this case, you need to determine if the practice or substance presents a danger to the patient. An example is the potential for interactions between certain herbal preparations and oral medications. Make the patient aware of these dangers if they exist.

Many home remedies have been handed down for generations and are quite safe. Trying to dissuade patients from this type of long-held belief may be viewed as disrespectful to their culture or families. You can convey respect for your patients' alternative practices by asking about the benefit that patients get from their use. You can also use this discussion to clarify any misconceptions.

47

I am uncomfortable when my patients bring product promotions for herbs, vitamins, and food supplements or indicate that they use alternative practices that I am not sure have any value. How can I deal with this in my DSME program?

 Tip

Acknowledging that you don't have firsthand knowledge about the effi-cacy of alternative practices is appropriate. If possible, ask patients for the source of their information. Many of the health claims are presented as a cure-all or a quick-fix designed to appeal to the consumer. The fact that the patient has brought the information to your attention indicates that he or she values your opinion.

Because both science-based and fiction-based health information is readily available from a variety of sources, we usually thank the patient for bringing the information to our attention and then investigate further. We share our findings and our sources with the patient. Some patients frequently bring us product claims, and their information stimulates us to stay current and contributes to a lively discussion in our diabetes group classes.

The great majority of alternative practices do not present a danger to patients. If patients perceive benefit from an alternative practice, there is no particular reason to discourage its use. However, encourage patients to test their perceptions empirically through frequent blood glucose mon-itoring so that they can make decisions based on evidence. Along with any effects on glycemic levels, alternative practices may help patients feel better and reduce the stress associated with diabetes. In this case, the patient's experience is the final determinant of whether that practice has value.

48.

I have some patients who have suffered significant vision loss. What can I do to ensure that my education program takes this problem into account?

 Tip

Educating a patient with vision loss can be challenging. Consider what content areas you need to teach differently. For example, modify lessons on drawing up insulin or using meters or other devices. Review the materials and teaching aids that you normally use, and try to determine which would be appropriate for someone who has low vision.

Other helpful strategies include the following:

- Use large-print materials with a minimum font size of 14. Ask your patients if the font size is large enough for them to read.
- Be sure that lighting in the room is sufficient. Add lighting or change rooms if necessary.
- Use light sticks or display lighting to illuminate key educational models or detailed diagrams. Have patients consider their lighting needs at home and work, and encourage them to make appropriate changes.

A great deal of communication is nonverbal. A patient with low vision can easily miss a nonverbal emphasis without the educator realizing it. When working with patients with visual impairments, we need to convey messages verbally that we usually convey nonverbally. For example, using strong vocal emphasis to make important points is more effective for these patients than using gestures or shifts in posture. Also, check frequently with patients with low vision to ensure that they understand you and that the information you are providing meets their needs.

49

I have had to repeat the same instructions to some of my patients at each visit. How can I tell if they have a hearing deficit?

 Tip

Patients suffering from hearing loss may

- lean close to you when you speak
- cup an ear with their hand
- speak loudly to you
- give inappropriate answers
- look blank when you speak to them
- seem inattentive or uninterested

Refer the patient to a hearing specialist for an assessment. If the patient is inappropriate for or unable to obtain a hearing aid, you will need to make accommodations in the way you teach.

50

I have noticed that a number of my older patients suffer from hearing loss. Do you have any advice about teaching patients with hearing impairments?

 Tip

Hearing diminishes with age and lifetime exposure to loud noises. If you obtain a physician's order, you may be able to receive reimbursement for teaching hearing-impaired patients individually rather than in a group.

Some helpful strategies include the following:

- Choose a quiet teaching space with little to distract attention away from your message.
- Minimize competing noises, such as a blowing fan in the cooling system, loud noises in an adjoining room, or multiple conversations in the same room.
- Help patients who read lips by arranging the room so the light will be on your face and not behind you.
- Speak in a lower—rather than louder—voice and face the patient.
- Speak clearly and slowly so that the patient can hear all of your syllables and ending letters.
- Prepare to use pictures, diagrams, and hands-on techniques to assist your teaching.
- Notice which way the patient turns his or her head regularly when you speak. That is likely the ear with the best hearing, so make sure you are on that side.
- Use short sentences to emphasize your point.
- Repeat yourself often or ask the patient to recite key information you have shared.

Tip *Continued*

- Use a gesture or transition to change your topic.

- Limit the number of topics covered at each session to avoid overwhelming the patient.

- Write down important points on a take-home sheet.

- Ask the patient what helps him or her learn something new. This question could be posed in future assessment forms to catch potential communication problems early on.

Adapted from Haas L: Education strategies for geriatric populations. *Today's Educator* 2(2):1–4, 2000.

B Bonus

How can I tell if my patients can afford the diabetes supplies and medications they need to take care of their diabetes?

 Tip

Caring for diabetes is expensive, and some people have difficulty paying for the supplies. As a first step, ask assessment questions such as, "Has caring for your diabetes created any financial problems for you?" or "Do you ever have a problem paying for your diabetes supplies?" or "Does your insurance cover your supplies and medications?"

Because many patients are hesitant to admit that they are having financial problems, you can look for some clues. For example, if patients stop monitoring their blood sugars or if their blood pressure has started to rise, cost may be an issue. At that point, you can ask patients why they are monitoring less or why their blood pressure is starting to rise. You can also ask if they are having difficulty paying for the strips or the medications. If a lack of money is the reason, they are often relieved that you asked these questions, especially if you offer resources that can help. Keep in mind that the loss of a job, the changing economy, or competing financial priorities can affect patients who were previously able to afford their supplies and medications.

Many of my patients have multiple needs. I know there are lots of resources out there. How do I find the resources my patients' need?

 Tip

Many patients have multiple needs, but there are usually a variety of resources available in your hospital and community. It can feel overwhelming to think that you have to provide information about all of them. Try narrowing your search by thinking about your typical patients and the type of resources they need most often. If you have a social work department in your facility, meeting with the staff and describing your target population is a good place to begin. Listings of available resources are often available from community health departments, state health departments, and local diabetes organizations. Specific options can include the following:

- Financial help is often available through referral to the social work department in your facility, the auxiliary or volunteer organization in your hospital, local churches, and charitable organizations such as the Lion's Club and Salvation Army.

- Scholarships for your education program can be solicited from private individuals, local businesses, and pharmaceutical and durable medical equipment companies in return for advertising.

- The social work department and community mental health clinics can help with family counseling and other psychological services.

- Meals-on-Wheels, home care, and other elderly support services can help patients remain independent.

- There are resources designed for special needs, for example, children or patients with complications from diabetes. The Internet, the yellow pages, or the community health department in your state often list these resources.

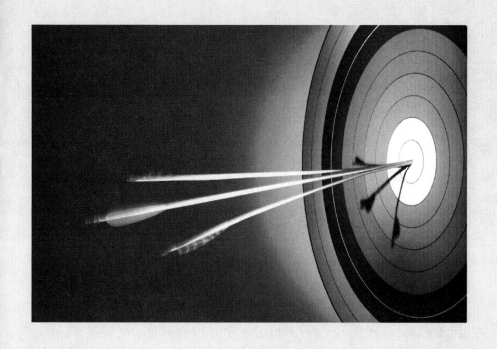

CULTURAL

COMPETENCY

51

I've heard that DSME should be culturally sensitive. What does this mean?

◎ Tip

Defined broadly, culture includes not only race or ethnicity but also a variety of other factors such as religion, socioeconomic status, gender, age, and geographic locale. All of these domains can be thought about as cultures that influence the way patients think about having and managing their diabetes

When working with a well-defined cultural group such as Native Americans, it is important that the educator, program, and program materials display sensitivity to and respect for that particular culture. Examples used in class and written materials need to portray and fit with that cultural group. However, the culture(s) of patients will often be neither obvious nor similar among participants in a group. In this case, examples used in class and written materials need to portray a variety of cultural groups.

52

Some of my patients are members of cultural groups that are different from my own. How can I assess cultural influences in a way that shows sensitivity?

 Tip

Culture is an important issue in diabetes that extends well beyond racial and ethnic groups to any group that shares common beliefs and traditions. Many cultural groups have beliefs and norms about health, illness, family roles, and health providers (which can include spiritual as well as clinical healers).

A useful way to assess cultural influences is to ask patients, "What cultural or religious practices affect how you care for your health or your diabetes?" Encouraging a discussion of these issues conveys respect for the role of cultural influences in patients' lives and in their diabetes self-management. The discussion can also help educators become more aware of the cultural influences that shape their patients' approach to self-management and often results in a group discussion that helps participants understand each other.

Also assess the patient's role in the family and the family's role in supporting (or, in some cases, not supporting) the patient's efforts at diabetes self-management. Do diabetes self-management recommendations put the patient in conflict with important family roles or cultural traditions? You can offer to work with these patients to adapt their self-management to fit with the important aspects of their culture and families.

A number of cultures view a variety of people other than traditional health care providers as sources of information and advice about health and illness. This can include elders in the family or community, medicine men or women, herbalists, and religious leaders. If your patients value advice from community elders, ask how patients combine that advice with diabetes self-management.

53

I have just begun providing diabetes care and education at a clinic that serves a cultural group other than my own. I want to adapt my diabetes education to my patients' culture. How can I learn about their cultural beliefs and traditions?

◎ Tip

Our approach is to use what some writers have called "cultural humility" as our touchstone. This means we start from the premise that all cultures, traditions, and practices are as deserving of respect as our own. Our patients can be wonderful teachers if we ask them questions and let them know that we are genuinely interested in their culture. Convene a group of patients and ask them how you can be sure that the education you provide is relevant to their culture. You could also ask those who attend your program to discuss some of their beliefs and practices related to health, illness, family roles, and religion. Visiting religious or other community centers or participating in celebrations and holidays can also help you learn a great deal about the culture and demonstrates respect and interest for the patients.

Other clinicians who have worked with these patients may be an important source of information as well. However, determine whether their attitude is one of compassion and respect or one of condescension before listening to their advice and guidance.

As educators, we need to help patients from all cultures minimize conflict with their cultural traditions and maximize the use of cultural resources to support their self-management efforts.

54

I believe that religion helps many of my patients cope with their diabetes. Is there an appropriate way to talk about religion during our DSME program?

 Tip

Religion and spirituality do in fact help a substantial number of patients cope with diabetes and a variety of other challenges in life. The culture of health care has become so scientific and secular that many patients feel that anything they say about religion or spirituality is unwelcome.

When we have introduced this topic during group classes, we have been surprised and gratified to hear how positively participants respond. To bring this topic up, we simply ask, "Does your religion or spiritual life help you cope with diabetes?" This question makes patients aware that talking about the support they get from their religious or spiritual practices is welcome in our education program and often leads to an animated discussion. Acknowledge to your patients the significant individual differences among people regarding religion, and state that you are not promoting any particular religion and that all practices and faith traditions will be respected.

55

I feel uncomfortable when my patients bring up religious or spiritual topics in our discussions. I know this is important to them and would like to become more comfortable. What advice can you give?

Tip

Health beliefs and spiritual beliefs are intertwined for many people. Patients will often provide clues that spirituality or religion is important to them by frequently referring to religious gatherings, readings, or events. This gives you a glimpse of the activities that may be a core part of your patient's lives.

Familiarity with a specific religion is helpful but not essential in assessing the role of spirituality in a patient's life and its impact on diabetes care. Ask the patient, "How do your religious or spiritual beliefs influence how you take care of yourself?"

Before you ask the question, determine if you can comfortably and effectively facilitate discussions of religion and spirituality even when the beliefs and practices differ from your own. Self-assessment questions could include:

- Do I have a strong belief that religion has its place, but not in health care?
- Do I dismiss discussions on spiritual topics because I see them as having no scientific basis?
- Do I become angry when religion is brought up?
- Because of my religious beliefs, would I be judgmental rather than supportive?
- Do I focus on the details of the religion rather than on the message of support that my patients derive from their beliefs?

If you answer yes to any of these questions, you may want to defer a discussion of religious topics until you have the opportunity to reflect further on these questions. You might also try talking with a coworker who has a different perspective of potential outcomes when including religion and spirituality in educational sessions.

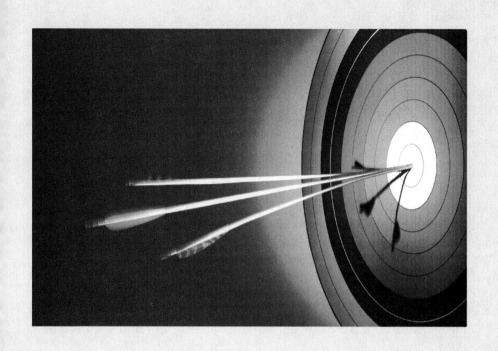

MEETING THE

NEEDS OF

SPECIAL POPULATIONS

56

__M__ore pediatric patients are coming to our practice and attending our classes. I am comfortable with adults, but I am not sure how best to work with children and teenagers.

 Tip

Working with children and teenagers means working with the whole family. Family members need to be included in diabetes education and management. Also, include family members in information gathering, but always direct some questions to the child once he or she is old enough to interact. As children grow older, begin asking them more questions. Because teens and parents may have different issues and concerns, they should each have time alone with the educator and the treatment team.

Get to know the child and family by having them describe what a typical day is like from the time the child gets up in the morning until he or she goes to bed at night. You are looking for a snapshot of their day—meal times, school routine, activities, and scheduling issues. You will then have the opportunity to explore the family's concerns and tailor treatment to their lifestyle.

For example, you may see a child who has gym the first hour at school and has trouble with low blood sugars before lunch. You can ask the family what strategies they have tried or believe will be effective to solve this problem. Offer options such as, "Would you like to have more food at breakfast, or would you rather lower your morning insulin dose on gym days?" Working with the family around specific issues teaches them how to incorporate diabetes self-management into their lives.

57

When teaching the family of a newly diagnosed child, there are so many competing needs and feelings. What is a good approach?

 Tip

At diagnosis, families are often overwhelmed with feelings of grief and with all the tasks they must learn to take care of their child. Start by providing the opportunity for them to talk about their feelings. Listen to and affirm those feelings. This is best done away from the child so parents won't need to worry about their child's reaction.

Families go through the grieving process and may experience intense feelings of anger, confusion, guilt, helplessness, disorganization, and denial. All of these reactions to the crisis of diagnosis are normal and may resurface at different times while living with diabetes. Allowing families to express negative emotions helps them mourn the loss of their healthy child and move forward in learning the skills necessary to manage diabetes.

58

Once I have helped families deal with the feelings related to the diagnosis of type 1 diabetes in their child, where do I start teaching so as not to overwhelm them?

 Tip

Focus on "survival skills" and "need to know" information when teaching newly diagnosed children and families. Set the stage—explain what will be taught and what the child and the family need to do. We have outlined our teaching plan for newly diagnosed families as follows:

C Carbohydrate counting—basics of carbohydrate counting

H Hypoglycemia—symptoms, management, and prevention

U Urine ketone testing—how to test and how to manage

M Monitoring blood glucose levels—how to check and record; determining targets

S Shots—how to draw up and give shots

Start where the patient is. Find out what he or she already knows. Help the patient break down management tasks and behavior changes into steps. When teaching skills, first explain, then demonstrate, and then have the patient and his or her family demonstrate the skill on themselves.

*W*hen teaching children and teenagers, who else needs to be included in the education?

 Tip

Two other involved individuals besides the child need to be instructed. The additional participants in diabetes education can be parents, step-parents, child care providers, grandparents, or other individuals who have responsibility for supervising and caring for the child.

The burden of responsibility for care should not fall on one individual's shoulders. Shared responsibility is essential to avoid burnout and ensure ongoing successful management.

Children, teenagers, and their families always need support and encouragement because they can't take a day off from diabetes. Parents need to stay involved and know the management plan even when their child or teenager is doing most or all of the self-management on his or her own. This allows parents to help with problem-solving and to take over injections or monitoring when their child needs a break or when their child is ill and needs help.

60

What resources would you recommend to families when their child with diabetes is having food issues?

 Tip

There are several excellent books available. One book that focuses specifically on food and parenting a child with diabetes is *Sweet Kids*. This excellent book by Betty Brackenridge, MS, RD, CDE, and Richard Rubin, PhD, CDE, outlines how to handle food and meal planning and keep the peace in a family with a child with diabetes. Using a developmental approach, the book offers many suggestions and strategies for the parent's role in diabetes care from infancy through adolescence.

Sweet Kids is published by ADA. ADA publishes many books for families with children with diabetes, including *Guide to Raising a Child with Diabetes, Real Life Parenting of Kids with Diabetes, Getting a Grip on Diabetes: Quick Tips & Techniques for Kids and Teens,* and *Getting the Most Out of Diabetes Camp: A Guide for Parents and Children.* All ADA books are available at http://store.diabetes.org.

*H*ow do I teach older children and teens about the complications of diabetes? I don't want to frighten them.

 Tip

We find it helpful to start by asking the group what they have heard about complications. After they share what they know, we ask, "How do these stories make you feel?" and allow time for them to share their feelings. It is important that parents attend or are aware of these discussions so they can feel reassured and help their child deal with this content.

Next we address what is known about diabetes complications. We share information from the DCCT and show how keeping blood sugars in or near the target range reduces the risk of complications. This information provides the rationale for giving three to four injections of insulin a day and for keeping A1C under 7% or 8%.

A body model allows us to show the kidneys, eyes, and nerves and discuss how they can be affected by elevated blood sugars over long periods of time. We discuss the goal of having a specific percentage (e.g., 75%) of blood sugar checks in the target range, and state that blood sugars may be higher during periods of rapid growth, stress, and illness. We teach kids how to make adjustments in insulin doses to lower blood sugars when they are outside the target range.

We explain why we check the blood pressure, measure growth, test A1C, and check their feet at every clinic/office visit. We also discuss why an annual blood draw for thyroid and cholesterol levels is needed and explain the purpose of the urine test for microalbumin. Let participants know that these checks are to help them prevent and detect the complications of diabetes.

Our discussion ends with a focus on the positive, such as new tools including new insulins, new meters, glucose sensors, new pumps, and the latest research in diabetes care. We encourage children and teens to learn all they can about diabetes so they can stay as healthy as possible until we develop better solutions for treatment or find a cure.

62

*A*re there important issues to consider when teaching a pregnant woman with diabetes?

 Tip

Yes. Besides the recommendations of the National Standards for Diabetes Self-Management Education, additional support and follow-up issues need to be addressed.

Managing diabetes is challenging for pregnant women. Support is particularly important during this stressful time. Suggest that they select a partner to support them in their daily diabetes care. Their partner will benefit from learning about insulin administration, food routines, the importance of blood glucose monitoring, the treatment of hypoglycemia and hyperglycemia, stress, emotional responses and needs, common discomforts, and emergency situations.

Issues to address with the expectant mother are

- fears and concerns about her health and the well-being of her infant
- expected weight gain
- care of other children during pregnancy and postpartum
- potential postpartum depression and how to recognize and manage it
- ongoing need for support
- postpartum care needs for her infant
- importance of follow-up care
- for a woman with gestational diabetes, address the importance of future screening, weight loss, maintenance, and physical activity to delay the possible onset of diabetes and the importance of facilitating health in her children

63

A *lot of older adults attend my DSME program. Are there specific things that I can do to make the sessions more effective for these participants?*

 Tip

Because diabetes is so common among older people, they are likely to make up a significant number of your DSME participants. Older adults are often very concerned about their health and eager to learn. As people age and experience chronic illnesses that threaten their independence, they often become more interested and able to take care of themselves than when they were younger and focused on working and raising a family. However, you must assess and accommodate the specific functional impairments that can occur as a result of aging.

Many older adults have multiple chronic illnesses, and diabetes may or may not be their most important consideration. Illnesses that affect them on a day-to-day basis may demand more of their attention. Provide information about diabetes in the context of other illnesses, and work with patients to incorporate various treatment programs into their daily lives. Older adults can make changes in their behavior and are often motivated by an awareness of how health contributes to their quality of life. Including significant others and family members has been shown to increase older adults' ability to learn and make behavioral changes.

D Bonus

I sometimes have caregivers of older adults in my classes. Are there specific ways that I can work effectively with them?

 Tip

Caregivers generally need the same type of personalized education and information that patients need. Some of the patients for whom they are caring may have different glucose and other goals than patients who can anticipate a long life with diabetes. You need to discuss these goals with the patient and his or her caregiver, physician, or other health care provider when appropriate.

Be aware of the limits that caregivers have. If the caregiver is the spouse of an older adult who is also elderly and has chronic illnesses, you need to accommodate their limitations and provide information about resources and support services. If the caregiver is an adult child or sibling, recognize that their efforts may be limited by other priorities in their lives, such as their own children, work, or families.

Along with providing information, it is important to recognize the toll that being a caregiver can take. Statements such as, "It must be really tough for you to manage your mother's diabetes and take care of your family," can help the caregiver feel supported and recognized.

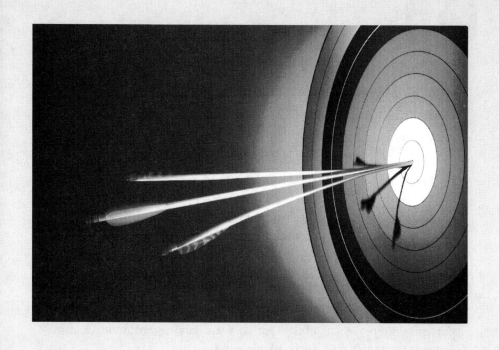

EDUCATIONAL

MATERIALS

64

I understand literacy is an issue in diabetes education. How will I know if my patients are struggling with literacy?

Tip

Literacy is the ability of an individual to read, write, speak a language, and compute or solve problems. Functional literacy is the ability to use these skills to meet the requirements of everyday situations. Health literacy refers to the ability to use these skills to participate in diabetes self-management and goal attainment. Because literacy is a continuum, individuals are rarely completely illiterate.

Patients often give us clues that they are having problems reading by making statements like, "I left my glasses at home," "My eyes aren't working right now," or "I have to go soon. Can I just take my paperwork home with me and send it back to you?" Other clues are looking blankly at the page and not following along when you refer to written materials.

Patients who repeatedly avoid or defer paperwork also alert us to their struggle to read, write, or comprehend written words. Patients who have language difficulties, such as newly immigrated patients with a limited ability to speak English, generally also have a limited ability to read English.

Low literacy does not mean an inability to learn. Patients with low levels of literacy learn well from concrete examples and repeated demonstrations. Ask all patients to repeat back important written information (e.g., prescription label instructions) and demonstrate skills.

I work in a community in which a high proportion of adults have low levels of literacy. How do I choose or develop appropriate educational materials?

 Tip

Ask yourself what are the most essential points about diabetes management and stick to those. Outlines with clear headings help you and the patient review the main points by using short, concise sentences and definitions. Decide what concepts need to be written, verbalized, or drawn to clarify important points. If you have assessment forms or questionnaires for participants to complete and you suspect or know that a patient reads poorly, offer to read the questions and write down his or her answers. You can also ask the patient if he or she would like to take the form home.

Select large-print, picture-based materials written at a third to sixth grade level based on SMOG or other reading tests. Choose written materials with simple words—the fewer syllables the better. Although you can't avoid words like diabetes and hyperglycemia, words that aren't specific for the content need to be as simple as possible. For example, use the word "get" instead of "develop," "pills" instead of "medications," and "shots" instead of "injections." Simply written materials still need to convey an adult tone.

Written materials for the low-literacy patient include

- a short, concise definition of the concept and a phonetic spelling of a difficult or uncommon key word (e.g., diabetes [di-a-bee-tees])
- a short, one- or two-sentence description of why the concept is important to the patient
- a picture or word picture that supports the concept
- key supportive points couched as action steps the patient can try

65

Tip *Continued*

Choose or develop written materials with adequate amounts of white space. White space makes the page uncluttered and less intimidating. Percentages, fractions, and decimal points are especially difficult. Bar graphs with simple text can be used to show proportional differences and express abnormal versus normal values.

People who don't read well often don't learn well from reading—even when you use materials with lower reading levels. A more effective method may be videotapes that patients can view in the classroom or take home. Another method is using commonplace models that illustrate difficult concepts. For example, explaining that pouring grease into a sink drain will eventually cause a clog illustrates the concept of a clogged artery. Another example is to compare our body cells to a room with a closed door. Insulin opens a door into the cell so that the glucose can enter.

Selecting or developing educational materials with the above points in mind will facilitate learning not only for your patients with low literacy but may also appeal to first-time learners of diabetes self-management.

66

What kind of print materials do patients usually prefer?

 Tip

Because adults prefer materials that get to the point quickly and emphasize important take-home messages, look for focused materials rather than comprehensive discussions of the clinical and scientific aspects of diabetes. In the past, print materials were often overly complex because of the concern that all relevant information be included. It's ironic that this approach, while providing more information, often actually impeded learning.

If your target audience is older or busy adults, look for materials with spaced text and lots of white space around key points. Younger people or people with lower levels of literacy may prefer stories presented as a photo novella or comic book with a lot of pictures and color and a small amount of text. Story formats are generally a powerful way to convey information to people of any age and any literacy level.

67

*T*here are so many excellent print materials
available. Do you have some advice about what
criteria (in addition to accuracy) I should use to
choose print materials for my DSME program?

 Tip

Print materials convey a tone. Materials written in a conversational
tone indicating respect for the intelligence of the audience are generally more effective than didactic materials (i.e., those that when read
aloud sound more like a lecture than a conversation) that just provide the
"dos" and "don'ts" without giving reasons. As you review the materials,
ask yourself if the materials are written in a way that will make the reader
feel talked down to or judged. If so, they will probably not be effective.

When you evaluate a document, compare its objectives with your own.
Are they similar or complimentary? Is the philosophy of the material
consistent in content and tone with your program's philosophy?

Consider the fit between the reading level of your target audience and
the reading level of your materials. For example, if you would describe
your target population as "the general population," then materials written at the sixth-grade level or lower would be appropriate. If your
patients have lower literacy levels than the general population, then print
materials at the third- to sixth-grade level are appropriate.

Look for materials with a good match between pictures and written
content. For example, a brochure about exercise is more effective with
photographs of adults engaged in physical activity such as dancing, walk-
ing, and swimming. Make sure the pictures match the ethnicity, age, and
body size of your audience.

68

There are a lot of print materials available for DSME. Are there any situations when you would recommend that I develop my own print materials?

 Tip

You're correct when you say that print materials are available in abundance. ADA, the American Dietetic Association, and many pharmaceutical companies have developed excellent print materials that can be used in DSME programs. Over the past ten years, companies have sought the help of diabetes educators in the development of print and audiovisual materials, and consequently their quality has improved substantially.

Even with the abundance of high-quality, low-cost (or free) materials, a few situations may prompt you to develop your own. For example, there may be key points in one or more of your lessons that you repeat several times during your oral presentations.

Although those points may be somewhere in existing print materials, they may not be highlighted and emphasized. A one- or two-page handout that summarizes these essential points and presents them in the same order as your presentation reinforces them visually to participants. A list of essential points separated by plenty of white space facilitates note-taking, which in turn promotes further reinforcement and personalization of the content.

Supplemental print materials may be useful when identifying resources specific to your community—for example, a list of foods that are particularly enjoyed by your audience with nutrition information about each food. Lists such as these can be used to supplement classroom presentations and discussions. Patients can keep the list with them as they are shopping for food or preparing meals. Although print materials can be an

68

Tip *Continued*

effective supplement to your instruction, each piece should be understandable, even to someone who hasn't attended your program.

An advantage to making your own handouts is that you can market yourself and your institution as the source of the materials by including the name of your program or logo. Be sure to copyright all of the materials you develop. Materials are copyrighted by simply indicating ©, your institution, and the year developed. For more information on copyright, visit the web site for the Office of Copyright at the Library of Congress (lcweb.loc.gov/copyright).

69

I work with specific populations and have decided to develop some of my own print materials. What steps should I take to ensure that the materials I develop are effective?

 Tip

Begin by choosing a group of expert consultants, that is, the participants in your classes. Because your patients will be using the materials, their insights and preferences are of great help in determining appropriate reading levels and sensitivity to educational and cultural needs. Show your patients available print materials and ask them what they like or dislike about each one. Then show them samples of the materials you have created and obtain the same feedback.

When you create sample materials, experiment with different fonts, formats, and pictures and have your patients indicate which ones they find most appealing. Consider using a particular style or format to convey your message to your target audience. Use desktop publishing software for a professional appearance. Possible formats include a comic book, Q & A, or testimonial. Report statistics with tables or graphs, and include a resource list.

To develop materials for a targeted population, consider including

- a definition of the problem or condition
- objectives of the brochure
- the relevance of the problem
- how to identify the problem
- actions to address the problem or identify the condition
- a list of local resources and information about your program

After you've gotten feedback from patients, ask coworkers, your program advisory committee, and/or your marketing department to review drafts of your print materials. Their feedback will ensure that you will have a high-quality product. Include copyright information and any restrictions on copies for use by the community or other professionals.

70

I have ideas for posters and handouts that I would like to make, but I'm afraid that next to professionally made materials mine will seem homemade. Do you have any thoughts about this issue?

 Tip

Production values are not the only determinant of the effectiveness of educational print media—most important is the extent to which patients can understand and relate to the material. Furthermore, your enthusiasm for the materials you develop will significantly increase their effectiveness because enthusiasm is contagious. Also, desktop publishing enables you to make your own materials and still have a professional look. Ask your colleagues and patients for their opinion about the appearance of these materials.

Materials you develop are likely to be a natural extension of the way that you teach and discuss diabetes self-management, therefore increasing the likelihood that you will use the materials as an integrated component of your teaching.

I've heard the saying, "A picture is worth a thousand words." Do you have any suggestions about how to get the most out of pictures, diagrams, or other types of illustrations?

 Tip

Many elements of diabetes patient education (e.g., words, pictures, and food models) are representations of some aspect of a patient's life with diabetes. Pictures, diagrams, and illustrations that closely represent the patient's experience will increase their effectiveness. For example, a written description of a meal is less effective educationally than food models. Food models are closer to the way the meal would actually be experienced by the patient and allow patients to use both visual and sensory modes to translate the message and to build a realistic meal.

Another example is to describe a biochemical process by using a body illustration that highlights an organ in its appropriate place rather than using a picture of an isolated organ. You could also have patients use their own body as a learning aid by instructing them to look at or feel the blood vessels in their hands, wrists, or neck as you talk about circulation.

72

I have a limited budget. Do you know of any inexpensive, simple visuals that I can use to teach nutrition?

◎ Tip

Two-dimensional food cards are inexpensive, easy to carry, and show correct portion sizes of food in realistic color. One type that can be purchased from the United Dairy Council includes information on the back that lends itself to carb counting activities and food label exercises. These can be purchased from the Dairy Council of Michigan, 2163 Jolly Road, Okemos, MI 48864; phone: (517) 349-8480, fax: (517) 349-6218; item number 0012NDC.

Plastic food models, though, have multiple advantages. They offer a more realistic representation of food. Models allow for handling, which is especially important for patients with vision problems. Although more expensive, plastic models last longer and do not become spoiled or torn. Nasco food models are available by calling (800) 558-9595 or by visiting www.nascofa.com/prod.

Food Guide Pyramids are by far the least expensive nutrition visual because master copies can be downloaded from the USDA Human Nutrition Information Service web site and photocopied. Food Guide Pyramids are becoming more common and can also be found on bread wrappers and cereal boxes. The web site from which to obtain these pyramids is www.usda.gov/cnpp/pyramid.htm.

All visuals have disadvantages as well. For example, the food cards are less effective than food models in representing portion size. Plastic food models frequently lack realistic color, which may make it difficult for patients to recognize the food that the model represents. Food Guide Pyramids group foods into unfamiliar categories and may not depict common foods for all ethnic groups. Because people often think of food as meals and snacks, single items promoted in the pyramid may make it harder for patients to apply these foods to their own meal plans.

I know that the effective use of videotapes facilitates learning. Do you have any specific advice about when to use videotapes in DSME?

 Tip

Design the beginning of each session to allow the participants and the educator to interact in a way that will facilitate subsequent participation and discussion. Therefore, as a general rule, a discussion or personal sharing is a better way to begin a session than showing a videotape.

During a session, videotapes can be used to break a longer presentation into shorter segments and to stimulate discussion. Videotapes are also a good way to introduce complex materials, such as insulin transporting glucose into cells. Participants will be able to better relate to the videotape if the people pictured resemble the audience in terms of age, gender, and ethnicity.

F
Bonus

__M__any of my patients now have access to the Internet, but they don't always get good information. What can I do to help them?

 Tip

More and more adults are computer literate, and older adults are the largest group of new Internet users. You can help them by recommending sites with reliable information.

Some reliable sites that also offer links to other good sites are listed in the table below.

Web site	Organization
www.diabetes.org	American Diabetes Association
www.aadenet.org	American Association of Diabetes Educators
www.cdc.gov/diabetes	Centers for Disease Control and Prevention (CDC)
www.ndep.com	National Diabetes Education Program (NDEP)
www.niddk.nih.gov/health/ diabetes/NDIC	National Diabetes Information Clearinghouse (NDIC)
www.niddk.nih.gov/health/ diabetes	National Institute of Diabetes and Digestive and Kidney Diseases (NIDDK)

There are other helpful web sites as well. For example, www.edhaynes. com includes interactions between herbs and prescription drugs and www. consumerlab.com is an independent lab that assays alternative treatments to verify dosages and check for contaminates. Pharmaceutical companies

Tip *Continued*

that provide patient education materials often have these available on their web sites as well.

To find other sites, just go to any search engine and search for "diabetes" or "diabetes education." Ask your computer-literate patients about sites they have found helpful. They may have found some good sites you don't know about. Be sure to check out these sites before recommending them. Ensure that the information is reliable. It may be useful to create a handout of dependable sites to give to patients.

Encourage patients to bring information they learn from the Internet to class or to their provider appointments. Remind them that if they are getting conflicting information from sites, you will be happy to look at both sites and discuss it with them.

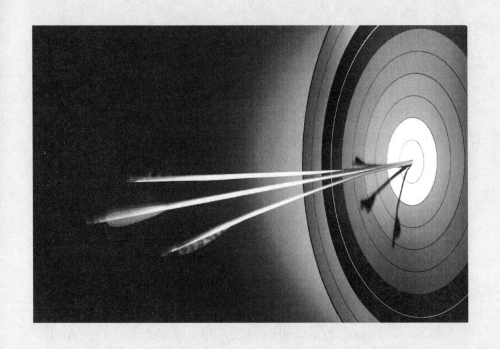

FACILITATING

GROUP SESSIONS

73

I've recently gone from teaching patients one-on-one to teaching group sessions. How can I make the group sessions as effective as the one-on-one sessions?

◎ Tip

Begin by thinking about what made your individual sessions effective. For many educators, it was the ability to personalize diabetes information and use the patient's experiences in the teaching process. Next, think about ways to incorporate these strategies into your group program. The key is usually to focus less on objective diabetes information and more on the participants' personal experiences with diabetes.

You can use these experiences even when teaching in a group. For example, when talking about hypoglycemia, you can ask, "Is there anyone here who has had hypoglycemia and would be willing to tell the group about it?" Questions you can use to add to the discussion are: "What symptoms did you have? What did you do? How did you feel afterwards? What do you think caused it? Did you have any particular kind of emotional response? What did you learn from the experience? Has anyone had a different experience with hypoglycemia?" You can then add to the experience and present additional content on the topic. Many patients are glad to share their experiences, and their stories make the content come alive for the rest of the group. Patients who are concerned about confidentiality will not volunteer their stories.

To help people become acquainted, increase group cohesiveness, and help participants feel connected to each other and the program, begin your program with icebreakers. Group activities or games can also help make classes more relevant and personal for each individual. You can do large or small group activities. If you have a large number of participants, divide the class into groups of three to five people to facilitate discussion and the sharing of problems and solutions. Suggest that each small group appoint a leader, but be sure that they choose a different one for each activity.

Do you know an effective icebreaker to use with a new DSME program series?

 Tip

There are a variety of effective icebreakers, and many educators have their personal favorites. A successful icebreaker is enjoyable, helps get people used to talking among themselves, and fosters relationships among group members and between the group members and the educator.

One icebreaker that we particularly like is having everyone in the group find one person that they do not know. Each member of the pair is given five minutes to introduce themselves to the other person. We encourage them not only to tell "diabetes diagnosis stories" but also to say some things about their work, recreational activities, family, or anything they think will help communicate who they are. After participants have had an opportunity to introduce themselves to their partner, we then go around the room, and everyone introduces their partner to the larger group. So, if John and Mary were paired, John would introduce Mary to the larger group. This activity is fun, helps people get to know each other, and fosters and reinforces the notion of listening carefully to the other members of the group.

75

Do you have any ideas about using homework to reinforce what is taught in my classes?

◎ Tip

To begin with, it is probably best to avoid the word "homework" because many people have negative feelings associated with this word from their days in school.

One strategy to help patients apply what they've learned is short-term goal-setting. Setting goals in class can be very effective. Although educators traditionally wait until the end of a series of classes to talk about and set goals, setting goals after the program is over will go more smoothly if you give participants the opportunity to practice along the way.

Present content about setting goals near the end of the first session. Ask participants to think of one thing that they could do before the next session that will help them take better care of their diabetes. Then, ask them to tell the group what their goal will be. Use your judgment about whether to call on those who choose not to state a goal. It is important that the behavior they choose is concrete, realistic, and truly their goal. They should be able to describe the when, where, what, how, and who of their goal. Suggest that they view the goal as an experiment, and tell them that they can discuss their experiences at the next session.

You can then begin each subsequent group session by having people report how their "goal experiments" went. They can discuss the results in the large group, as paired-sharing, or in groups of four to five people, depending on what will work best for your audience. Although not every patient will choose to participate, these experiences often provide rich topics for the entire group to discuss. When a patient's experiment doesn't go as planned, asking "why" is a way to help the patient learn from the experience without feeling judged.

At the end of each class, repeat the sequence of having people think of one more behavioral goal until the next class, and continue goal-setting each week until the end of the series. Once the series is over, patients can set goals independently or in collaboration with the educator.

I am just beginning a group DSME program.
Are there ground rules I can suggest to the group
to enhance the involvement of all participants
and in general make my classes run better?

 Tip

Explicit ground rules almost always improve group interaction and facilitate involvement by the widest number of participants. Ground rules that are public and agreed upon by all participants create a safe environment for individuals to speak up. Some of the ground rules we typically use in our group sessions are as follows:

- Only one participant talks at a time, and that person is allowed to finish before another participant speaks up.

- What works for one person may not work for another, so we respect individual differences of how people manage their diabetes.

- We encourage responsible communication by the frequent use of the word "I." For example, "I have learned . . ." or "In my experience . . ." as opposed to having group members make absolute statements about what is or isn't true.

- We ask participants to agree that what's said in class stays in class so that people can feel safe revealing things they might not reveal in a conventional social situation.

- The group facilitator may sometimes have to interrupt a participant so other participants can speak or so a new topic can be introduced.

You can write the ground rules on a flip chart and invite discussion on each rule. Ask the group to think about items that could be removed or added. At each subsequent group session, display the rules so members will be reminded of their commitment. Rather than inhibiting discussion, well-crafted rules increase both the functioning and the morale of the group.

77

*D*o you have any suggestions for encouraging class members who are quiet to participate more actively? Calling on them only seems to make the problem worse.

◎ Tip

The first question to address is if this is a problem for the participant or for you. Some people are quiet in a group setting because they learn best by listening. They can be fully engaged and still remain quiet. It is important to recognize and respect individual differences.

Other participants are shy and may want to speak but hesitate to do so. It may take them longer to begin to speak, and more assertive members may talk before they have an opportunity. Taking time to ask if anyone else has anything to add may give them the opportunity they need. Pay attention to their body language. If they look like they are ready to speak, you could say, "Mrs. Jones, would you care to add something?" before moving to the next topic or responding to another person.

Another strategy that has proved successful in other types of groups is to assign the quiet participant what are known as "power roles." This can be any task that helps single the person out in a non-threatening way and helps them feel like, and be viewed as, having an important role in the class. For example, ask the person to help you by handing out or collecting papers, writing ideas on a flip chart during a brainstorming session, or doing any other task that supports the work of the group. Although such activities may seem minor, they can have a significant impact on the perceived role and status of someone who may feel intimidated or alienated from the group.

78

How can I deal with nonstop talkers who make it difficult for other class members to participate?

◎ Tip

This can present a challenging situation, even for experienced educators, because it calls for behavior that in other situations would be considered impolite. At the beginning of class, acknowledge that as the facilitator you are responsible for maximizing the participation of all class members. State at the onset that you may need to interrupt someone in order to draw other members into the discussion. Be clear that such interruptions do not imply that you are displeased with the person you interrupt, but rather that you are committed to making sure that everyone has the opportunity to participate.

Then do it—interrupt the nonstop talker with a polite "Thank you, I appreciate your contribution, and now I would like to hear from some of the other members of the class." This can be uncomfortable because we have been taught that interrupting others is impolite, but if we do not act, we lose the goodwill and interest of the other class members who expect us to function as the group leader.

79

How do I deal with a person in a group who wants to offer everyone else advice on their problems?

 Tip

One strategy is to set the stage from the very beginning. During the introductions, tell participants that you encourage each person to develop their own solutions. Outline ground rules such as respect for each person, confidentiality, and allowing each person the opportunity to speak. You can also model ways to offer ideas by saying things such as, "Other patients I have known with this problem found that _____ worked for them. Do you think that idea will work for you?" You might point out that everyone is different and that what works for one individual doesn't necessarily work for another.

But sometimes, in the heat of the moment, a participant will blurt out: "Well you should . . ." or "Oh no, that's not what you're supposed to do!" At that point, one approach is to ask the person the comment is directed toward what he or she thinks of the advice. You can also ask the group for other suggestions or options and start a brainstorming session. At several points, ask the participant with the issue what he or she thinks of the various ideas.

If this type of behavior continues, talk with the person after class. Explain that your approach is to encourage individuals to develop their own strategies to deal with diabetes, and while you appreciate that his or her particular method has worked for him or her, there are other ways of meeting a similar challenge.

I have realized lately that I do not wait long enough after asking a question for someone in class to come up with an answer. I am having trouble breaking this habit. Can you offer any suggestions?

 Tip

This is a common problem in social as well as educational situations. Most educators wait about one second after asking a question before they answer it themselves, ask another question, or move on to present more content. On average it takes learners about three to five seconds to formulate an answer to a question. This means we need to pause at least three to five seconds after asking a question.

One technique that usually proves effective is to recite a nursery rhyme (in your head) after asking a question. For example, you could say to yourself "Mary had a little lamb, its fleece was white as snow, and everywhere that Mary went, the lamb was sure to go." This mental exercise will create the necessary three- to five-second pause, allowing class members to respond to the question. In a relatively short period of time, the nursery rhyme will be unnecessary because waiting three to five seconds for a response will become second nature to you.

81

I don't know how to respond when there are extended periods of silence during our class discussions. Do you have any advice on keeping a discussion going?

 Tip

You are right. Extended silences in a group that has been talking are often a real challenge to an educator because it is not possible to know for certain what the silence means. When we don't know what the silence means, it is difficult to know how to respond. If the participants are bored, we might respond one way, whereas if they are confused, we might respond another.

The best solution to this dilemma is to attack it head on. Say to the class, "You will have to help me understand what this silence means. I need to know whether you are bored or confused, or you've said all you want on the topic so I can respond in a way that will meet your needs." Then wait for an answer. There is almost always at least one person who will let you know what the silence is about.

82

A lot of my patients like to tell their stories about diabetes in class. How can I respond to these so that they are useful educational activities?

◎ Tip

Using patients' experiences can be tricky. Some participants may find that listening to others' positive experiences is beneficial, but participants who are struggling may find that such stories decrease their feelings of self-efficacy and make them feel less able to take care of themselves. Although other participants can perhaps relate to negative experiences, they leave the educator in a difficult dilemma of how to respond.

One of the ways to use these experiences is to ask patients to describe what they learned from what happened to them. Questions can include the following:

- What was the result?
- What did you learn about yourself? . . . about diabetes? . . . about others?
- What will you do differently next time?

These questions are appropriate and useful whether the behavior was positive or negative because they eliminate judgments. While the specifics of the examples may not be useful for the other participants, the experience and learning of a classmate may help them gain some insight into their own situation.

G Bonus

By the time I finish a series of diabetes education classes, the group has bonded and connected with each other on a personal level. This seems to happen so close to the end of the program that I feel participants miss out. How can I facilitate bonding and a sense of belonging earlier?

 Tip

People most commonly affiliate around perceived similarities. The fact that you are teaching people with diabetes and/or people close to them provides a good beginning. If the participants in your group sessions share other important similarities—for example, the same age-group or cultural group—facilitating camaraderie and connections is easier.

Establishing ground rules that support mutual respect may help the group connect on a personal level earlier in the process. One of the ground rules in our classes is that we respect each person's approach to diabetes self-management no matter how it may differ from our own. This ground rule may seem to emphasize differences, but in fact individual differences grow out of an underlying commonality. For example, when two patients describe the help they receive from others, one might describe receiving help and support from a friend, while another might focus on the help received from a spouse. This gives the educator an opportunity to point out that although they are receiving social support from different people, both patients recognize the importance of social support.

Sometimes surface differences represent underlying commonalties. For example, patients of different religions may both value their faith as a way to cope with diabetes. Also, patients who take very different approaches to self-management may share a commitment to doing the best job they can to manage their diabetes.

Tip *Continued*

There are also a number of specific techniques that facilitate the development of group camaraderie. Placing chairs in a circle or having patients sit around a table facing each other facilitates eye contact and promotes patient-to-patient interaction rather than just patient-to-educator interaction. Name badges or name tents allow people to address each other by name. Interactive assignments and discussions within the group also facilitate this process. Be on the lookout for members who seem hesitant to participate, and invite them to share experiences and join in activities.

Key behaviors of the educator that promote a connection are sitting with the group instead of in front or behind a desk. Make sure people have been introduced to each other. To increase name familiarity, we tend to use the names of members when we respond to their questions. Lastly, point out the similarities of experiences and strategies of the group members.

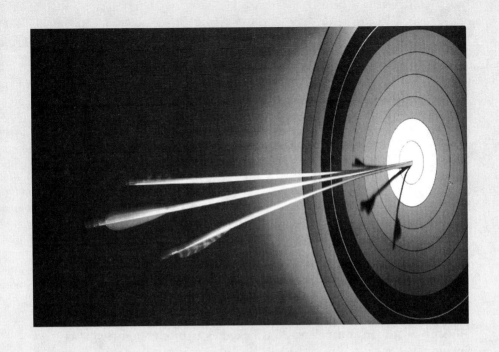

ENHANCING

TEACHING SKILLS

83

I've read that as educators, we need to recognize the patients' expertise. Does that refer to the post-test?

 Tip

Not really, although the post-test may measure what the patients have learned during the education part of the program. Recognizing our patients' expertise means respecting and valuing their knowledge about diabetes as much as we want our patients to respect and value our knowledge of diabetes. Patients' knowledge encompasses their priorities, circumstances, and experience with diabetes and problem-solving.

Recognizing the patient's expertise also means creating an equal partnership based on mutual respect. Diabetes is often the first experience many patients have with a chronic illness that requires extensive self-care. For most, this means establishing a different type of relationship with their health care provider. Although we expect this of patients, we don't often include a discussion of the roles and relationships needed for effective diabetes care as part of their education.

In our first session with a class or with individuals, we spend some time talking about our respective roles and the need to collaborate. We tell them that although we know about diabetes, we don't know about their lives. Each of us is an expert about our own lives. They are the experts on what will work for them. When we combine what we know with what they know, we make a powerful team.

84

I have been told that I should capitalize on teachable moments. What does this mean exactly?

◎ Tip

Generally, the term "teachable moment" refers to events that can result in a significant shift in the patient's perception of diabetes and diabetes self-management and provide significant motivation for learning more about diabetes. A teachable moment often happens when the patient has an "Aha!" as the result of an experience, but can also be facilitated by educators. As an example of the former, one of our patients told us that she was playing with her grandchildren one day when she realized how much she wanted to see them grow into adults. This realization changed her formerly lackadaisical attitude about her diabetes self-management and provided her with significant motivation to learn more about diabetes and apply that knowledge to her life. In this example, the patient capitalized on her teachable moment by seeking diabetes education.

Examples of opportunities to facilitate this type of teachable moment can occur during monofilament testing or while reviewing lab values. It is generally not possible to cause teachable moments, but we should be on the lookout for them and capitalize on them when they occur. Patients who have just learned that they are developing complications may be very open to learning more about diabetes. An educator can have a major impact on such patients. We can also facilitate and create opportunities for changes in perception by asking patients to reflect on what they are doing, what results they are getting, and their level of satisfaction with these results.

85

I have a noticed that some of the participants in my DSME program start to tune out of my lectures after about 15 or 20 minutes. Do you know any strategies for keeping them interested and engaged?

 Tip

A great many people lose interest after listening passively to a 15- or 20-minute lecture. One way to help participants pay attention is to introduce an activity designed to get learners actively involved every 10 or 15 minutes during your presentation. Such activities do not have to take a great deal of time—one or two minutes is usually enough. For example, after 10 or 12 minutes of a discussion, you can ask patients to write down the three most important take-away points from your presentation so far, and then have them share with someone sitting next to them. After about 2 or 3 minutes of sharing, you could ask how many of the participants' three take-away points exactly matched their partners. Other strategies are to have participants complete and discuss a work-sheet or case study related to the topic or to conduct a verbal quiz every 10 or 15 minutes on the materials just presented.

The important principle is that you want to give patients a chance to interact with and apply the information so that it will be retained.

86

I'm worried that many of the participants forget a lot of what I teach shortly after my DSME program ends. Do you have any suggestions for helping them retain the information longer?

 Tip

One technique (used at Harvard University*) that allows everyone in a large group to discuss key concepts lends itself readily to diabetes education. Identify the key concepts you wish to reinforce during the class and develop a true or false or a multiple-choice question for each key concept. Take a brief pause about every half-hour during your lecture to present one of the questions to the entire class, and ask each class member to write down what he or she believes to be the correct answer. Keeping the question and possible answers in full view during this exercise is helpful to the participants.

Next, invite the participants to turn to the person sitting next to them and spend 60 seconds discussing their answers. If the participants disagree, encourage them to try to convince the other person that he or she is correct. This exercise, which only takes one or two minutes each time, allows everyone in the class to interact and to think about what they know and why they believe it to be true. The activity has been shown to increase participant knowledge and the degree of confidence they have in their mastery of the information.

*Thinking Together: Collaborative Learning in Science (video). The Derek Bok Center for Teaching and Learning, Harvard University, Cambridge, MA, 1992.

87

I have my content presentations down pat, but they feel a little stilted. Do you have any suggestions for loosening things up a bit?

Tip

The stilted feeling you are referring to often occurs when the educator is paying more attention to the material than to the audience. A good way to loosen up a presentation and make it less formal is to begin to interact with the audience early on during the session. There are a variety of ways to do this, and you can choose those that seem appropriate to your style and your situation. For example, instead of standing behind a podium, sit or approach people, make frequent eye contact, and pay close attention to the expressions on participants' faces to see whether they appear confused or bored, or have missed a point. These behaviors help develop and maintain a psychological connection with your audience. Using techniques to help you establish a relationship with your audience will transform your educational sessions so that they will start to feel like conversations.

88

I have heard some speakers make their presentations more enjoyable through humor. How can I use humor to improve my classes?

 Tip

It depends. Humor is an effective teaching strategy only if it comes naturally and easily to you. A person who does not have the ability to tell humorous anecdotes should forego them altogether. An education session containing no humor is far better than an education session filled with failed humor.

That said, there are a number of useful goals that humor can help us achieve if it comes naturally to us. First, self-deprecating humor can help close the gap between teacher and participants and make the educator seem more human and accessible. A witty anecdote revealing one of the foibles of an educator can make that person seem "more like one of us" to the rest of the class. Humor, like crying, is also a form of release. From time to time, we all need some release, especially when dealing with a serious issue like diabetes. Also, laughter is a shared experience that can help members of the class overcome social distance and foster relationships. Finally, an amusing anecdote about a person's experience with diabetes self-management may help participants remember the educational content more easily.

However, humor can be used to harm or humiliate people. All of us can probably remember a painful incident as schoolchildren in which we were made fun of by other children. Because humor has both the power to help and to harm, it needs to be used compassionately and gently.

89

I've tried to have discussions in my class about patients' diabetes care priorities, but they seem kind of flat. Do you have any suggestions about making such discussions more lively?

Tip

We developed a technique that has been very successful in making discussions about patients' priorities lively and interesting. It is called the Values Auction. Make a list of ten or twelve priorities that you expect to be meaningful to patients with diabetes. For example, "Receiving care by a doctor who's interested in and knowledgeable about diabetes" or "Strong support from my family and friends in caring for my diabetes." Each priority on the list should be something that's both possible and relevant for people with diabetes. We print each priority on a 3 × 5 (or 5 × 7) card and then print copies with the entire list numbered one through ten or twelve.

Prior to the auction, we have the participants review the entire list. We then tell them we are going to auction off each one of the items on the list. We encourage the group to express the importance of a particular item by bidding on it. We give each patient $10,000 in play money for the bidding. We start with item number one and conduct the activity like a typical auction. Patients generally find the auction enjoyable. At the end, we ask each person who bid successfully for an item on the list to tell why that item is important to him or her. We also include participants in the discussion who tried to purchase that item but were outbid. Sometimes people purchase an item they don't have because they would like it, and other times participants purchase items that they do have to express how strongly they feel about their value.

90

When I ask questions in class to assess how much people know (e.g., "Who can tell me what causes a low blood sugar reaction?"), people often seem reluctant to answer. Any suggestions?

 Tip

Most of us do not want to appear ignorant in front of our peers. It is very natural to be reluctant to answer a knowledge-based question—which is really a form of an oral quiz—in public. However, we can rephrase such questions or change them entirely to make them less threatening. For example, asking people what they've heard about low blood sugar reactions is less threatening than asking them what they know. Another strategy is to ask people what they need to know more about or want to learn about a topic. This strategy allows class members to reveal what they don't know in a way that is not embarrassing.

91

I am uncomfortable with silence. Are there times when silence is a good thing during diabetes education?

Tip

Silence can be a very potent communication and relationship-building tool and can be effective in a variety of situations. For example, when we ask patients a question, silence makes it clear that we are comfortable giving them time to think about how they want to answer. This is likely to improve the quality of both the answer and our relationship. Also, if a patient has expressed a very strong emotion and/or described a very intense experience, simply sitting in silence for a few moments is a way of expressing respect for the significance of that communication. Finally, silence can be used as a brief rest or a respite from a challenging encounter.

In an overall sense, the more we offer our patients respectful silence, the more likely they are to fill that silence with important information about themselves and their experience of living with diabetes.

92

Do you have any advice about how and when to use stories in diabetes education?

 Tip

Yes. Stories are one of the most effective and powerful educational methods known. This probably explains why they have been around since the beginning of recorded history. Stories are universal because they are how we represent our experiences to ourselves and to others.

There are two basic ways to use stories effectively in diabetes education. One involves moving outward *from* the patient; the other involves moving inward *toward* the patient. For example, having patients tell their own stories in class is an example of the former. Patients telling their own stories can help a group bond and provides useful information to other members of the class. Furthermore, when patients tell their own stories, they often have insights into their own situations simply by listening to themselves describe their experiences.

The second way to use stories is to take information that may be essentially dry, clinical, scientific, or technical and incorporate it into stories that illustrate its importance and/or use. For example, stories from other patients you have known or stories that relate symptoms of diabetes to its pathophysiology move the content toward the patient. This strategy makes clinical information feel more relevant, practical, and human to the patients who are listening to and discussing these stories.

H Bonus

My son told me his English teacher said that analogies and/or metaphors can enhance teaching and learning. Does this apply to DSME?

 Tip

Analogies and metaphors are images or descriptions of the familiar used to represent the unfamiliar. The classic example in diabetes education is the use of keys to represent insulin unlocking cells to allow glucose to enter. Metaphors and analogies can be very powerful teaching tools because they allow people to grasp the unfamiliar by comparing it to something that is well known to them.

For example, when patients in our class ask whether lower blood glucose levels prevent complications, we of course have to answer that it would reduce their risk but that there are no guarantees. A metaphor that has worked very well is to ask people to imagine they are at a social event and need a ride home. Two friends offer them a ride—one who has been drinking to excess and another who is sober. When asked who they would choose to ride home with, people invariably chose the sober driver. We then ask, "Does riding home with someone who is sober guarantee that you won't get into an accident?" They usually say "No." We ask, "Does riding home with someone who has been drinking guarantee that you will get in an accident?" "No," they say. Then we ask, "Why choose the sober driver?" We use this analogy to talk about the risk reduction benefits of lower blood glucose in a world in which there are no guarantees.

The best way to evaluate the usefulness of a metaphor is to pay careful attention to how patients respond to it. Do they understand it immediately? Can they relate to it on a personal and emotional level? Does it facilitate and enliven a subsequent discussion of the issue? Just as beauty is in the eye of the beholder, the effectiveness of a teaching strategy lies in the response of the learner.

I have heard that role-playing can be used as part of DSME. Do you have any advice about when or how to use it?

 Tip

Role-playing can be a powerful educational strategy when used skillfully. To facilitate role-playing, the educator needs to have good interpersonal skills and be comfortable leading a discussion about psychosocial issues (i.e., emotional aspects of diabetes; relationships with family, friends, and health professionals; or behavior change).

One very effective use of role-playing is a behavioral rehearsal. If a patient needs to have a potentially uncomfortable conversation with a family member or caregiver about some highly charged issue, practicing the conversation using role-playing exercises can be excellent preparation for the actual event. Another scenario where role-playing can be effective is when a patient is dissatisfied with some aspect of medical care but is uncomfortable bringing it up for fear of alienating his or her provider. The patient can practice ways to introduce the topic so the likelihood that the physician will be offended is minimized and the patient remains true to his or her feelings.

Role-playing another person's point of view is also a good way to deepen one's empathy. Using the previous example, we might say, "I'll role-play you, and you role-play your provider to see how she might respond when you bring up your issue." Successful role-playing requires a fairly high degree of trust among the members of the group as well as an educator who is skilled and comfortable in dealing with emotions.

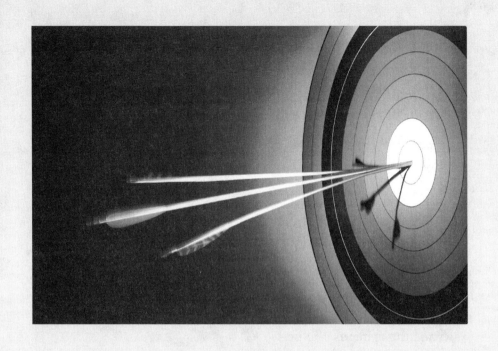

CHALLENGING

PATIENTS

93

The participants in my education program have often heard incorrect information about diabetes from other sources. How can I convey my expertise so that they believe that I am competent?

 Tip

Competence is an important quality to convey because it influences how much we will put our faith and trust into another person's hands. How do you decide that people you encounter are competent? We often form opinions based on the level of confidence the person projects, his or her education or experience in the area, his or her affiliation and role, and the opinions of others.

Here are some tips that will help you to convey your expertise:

- Present the information confidently and correctly.
- Acknowledge when you don't know the answer to a question. Most people can tell when you are not sure because your confidence level changes.
- Describe your role, special training, and background in diabetes education.
- Humanize yourself by offering some personal information.
- Acknowledge the patient's expertise in living with diabetes. Knowing about diabetes and knowing about another person's diabetes are not the same thing.
- Use data. Statements such as, "The latest research shows" and "Here's what I know about . . ." help people to evaluate the quality of the information.
- Convey empathy and caring. Most people look for health care providers who are not only competent, but who are also caring.

94

How do I tell a patient what he or she knows about diabetes is incorrect?

 Tip

It depends on the setting and the situation. First, you need to use a great deal of tact so that you don't embarrass the person who offered the information. This is true regardless of the setting, but is particularly sensitive in a group.

The situation also has an impact. If you know the patient's information is incorrect, explain the correct information. You can preface it by a statement such as "We used to think that, but now we know . . ." or "I don't think that's completely true . . ." Offering articles or other corroborating evidence may be helpful. If patients stick with their beliefs, ask them where they heard their information or what led them to believe it is true.

Sometimes there is a link between truth and fiction. This happens with "old wives tales," where there is often a factual basis. Discuss what part is true and how one might then make incorrect assumptions.

Misinformation that sounds scientific or offers "scientific proof" can be harder to counter. Many stories that have no basis in fact circulate on the Internet or among people with diabetes. Offer evidence to the contrary, explain why the "science" is flawed, and offer alternative information supported by scientific data.

95

I don't know how to respond when participants in a class give wrong information to the group. What do you suggest?

 Tip

Responding to this situation is difficult because you don't want to discourage participation or embarrass the person who made the statement. However, you have several options. If the information is incorrect and potentially harmful, it is important and appropriate to respond. The following statements may help to depersonalize and defuse the situation.

- "My experience is . . ."
- "Here's what I know about that . . ."
- "You may have found that effective, but everyone is different . . ."
- "There really isn't evidence to support . . ."

Other statements such as, "I've never heard about that. Let me do some checking, and I'll tell you what I find out at the next class," is another way to respond to the situation. If you can provide evidence that the information is wrong, try using a statement such as, "Let's think about that for a minute," before giving the correct information. This strategy was useful to us when a participant told the rest of the class that honey in lemon juice was a good treatment for high blood sugar.

If the information does not really matter, it may be best to not respond. For example, we chose not to respond when a participant informed the rest of the class that type B blood was generally thicker than the other types.

96

*S*ometimes I am asked questions and I don't know the answer. What should I say?

◎ Tip

It is always difficult when you are not sure what the answer is to a patient's question. Being able to admit that you don't know the answer is a sign of maturity as an educator. Diabetes is a very complex chronic illness, and there isn't always one correct answer—there may be several.

If you are asked a question you can't answer, simply say you will find the answer and bring it to the next class. You might try one of the following responses:

- "I will have to check on the answer to that question; I am not quite sure."
- "That is a good question, but I don't have the answer. I will have to get back to you."
- "Let's check with the other team members and see if they know."

97

I've taught a few classes in which patients seem to know more about a particular diabetes-related topic than I did. This made me very uncomfortable because I thought the class would doubt my competence as an educator. What would you recommend I do in such a situation?

 Tip

Almost all of us encounter patients who know more about particular topics than we do. A skilled educator is a good communicator. Our role is more than just a repository and transmitter of diabetes information. We not only provide information, but we also facilitate learning by using a variety of teaching and learning methods.

Everyone in your program is an expert on what works best in their lives. So, one way to head off the "expertise" problem is to begin the first class by acknowledging that the room contains a group of experts and that we all contribute to the education of the entire group.

If participants have expertise in a particular area, acknowledge and thank them for the contributions they make. However, even when acknowledging their expertise, be sure to listen carefully to what they say and clarify misinformation if necessary. Approaching education with an attitude that says, "We're all in this together, and we are going to help each other" will reduce the likelihood that you will feel this kind of discomfort.

98

Sometimes I do all the talking when a patient comes to see me, especially if I think that I have a lot to cover. How can I make the best use of the time we have together?

 Tip

It's easy to talk too much when you want to be sure that you have covered everything or when patients have a lot of needs. Ask yourself, "Whose needs are being met when I do this?" The next time you find yourself doing all of the talking, try this experiment: only ask questions. In our experience, this strategy helps us stay focused on the patient and produces some of the most productive educational sessions we have had.

Even though patients come to us to learn about diabetes, both patients and educators need to know how to fit diabetes into their lives. The patients are the ones who know the answers to those questions. Try the question experiment the next time you are with a patient. You'll be surprised at how much you both learn.

99

In almost every group class that I teach, one or two participants seem withdrawn. From observing their body language and listening to the few things they do say, I'm worried that they may be depressed. I wonder whether being in my class is doing them any good. Do you have any thoughts about this?

Tip

Signs of depression can include feigned interest or frank disinterest indicated by poor eye contact, unwillingness to ask questions or join in group discussions, and sitting in a way that is physically removed from the rest of the group. When depressed participants do speak, they may apologize for being distracted or express chronic pessimism about diabetes. Most depressed patients feel isolated and cut off. They can feel alone and alienated even when in group situations.

Depression is a barrier to learning in many ways. For example, many depressed patients recycle thoughts about the hopelessness of their situation and seldom have the energy for significant behavior changes. There are a couple of ways to deal with this problem. One is to discuss depression in class because it is such an important issue for people with diabetes. During the discussion, you can make salient points about how to tell if you're depressed and about the fact that there are effective treatments. Today, people don't have to simply put up with being depressed. Have literature about depression available for participants to take home so that they can become more familiar with this illness.

Another strategy is to take these participants aside before or after class and simply tell them that you're worried about them and offer a referral for a formal evaluation for depression. Express your willingness to initiate the necessary steps. Many depressed patients are unable to take the first steps to get treatment because they feel too hopeless. They will likely be grateful for your help.

100

I have referred my depressed patients for therapy, and thankfully, they are receiving it. How can I ensure that my diabetes education complements the therapy they are receiving for depression?

 Tip

Depression and diabetes go hand in hand and their treatment needs to also. For example, make sure there are no interactions or potential contraindications between their diabetes medications and antidepressants. Review the side effects of both types of medications with patients and their families.

In addition:

- Patients may experience weight changes with depression or from the medications. This can have an impact on their blood glucose levels. Discussing the potential for weight loss or weight gain ahead of time can prepare patients and help them prevent or deal with the changes.

- Support and reinforce your patients' decision to seek therapy. Medications for depression can take several weeks to show any benefit, and patients may need support to continue.

- Try matching the complexity and density of your education to the degree of improvement in your patients' depression. Avoid overwhelming patients with too much information while they are still depressed. Focus on survival skills.

- It can be useful to discuss blood sugar fluctuations related to the stress caused by depression.

Overall, the two major goals are to support their decision to seek help for their depression and to tailor your diabetes education to the amount of interest and motivation they have available for these tasks at any given time.

1

I know that some of my patients are not being candid with me when I ask them how things are going with their self-management plan, especially diet and exercise. How can I let them know that I appreciate honesty?

Tip

A good way to begin addressing this problem is to think about why people are not truthful. There is generally one cause: fear. People usually lie or withhold information in order to protect themselves from some perceived threat. In health care, patients are often less than candid when they are trying to avoid blame or criticism, either direct or implied, from the health professional. They may feel guilty about their inability to use some aspect of their management plan and are trying to avoid getting lectured or scolded.

If this seems to happen often, it may be worthwhile to reflect on your approach. Is it possible that your patients are worried that they will somehow be made to feel like they are failing or are inadequate? If so, are their fears grounded in reality or not? If your approach is maternal and you convey disappointment to your patients for what you perceive as inadequate self-management, then you can expect this behavior to continue. If on the other hand, you do not judge or try to get your patients to change, then perhaps the explanation lies with experiences they have had with other health professionals.

If the latter is the case, let your patients know that your approach to diabetes care and education is different. It may be worthwhile to have a discussion about the fact that you are not interested in having them care for their diabetes in order to win your approval, but rather your goal is to help them think about the relationship of their choices to their goals. You can reassure them that no matter what they tell you about their self-management, they will not be blamed or criticized. Establishing trust may take a series of visits, but in the end, it will increase the likelihood that the diabetes care and education you provide will be effective.

*I find it frustrating to work with patients
who don't seem to make diabetes care a high
priority. Any suggestions?*

 Tip

This frustration often comes from our need for patients to take care of their diabetes the way we think they should. The decisions that patients make are usually intended to help them meet their own needs, not ours. The solution lies in reflecting on and discovering the reason(s) we need patients to make diabetes care a high priority. Do we feel responsible for the choices they are making? Are we worried that they will develop complications and that somehow we will be at fault? Are we worried that we will be viewed as poor educators if our patients don't comply?

It's not wrong or unusual to want our patients to do their very best. However, it is important to realize when and if our behavior is a reaction to our need for patients to change rather than their need to change. If we are frustrated with patients because we need them to change, our frustration will be communicated to them in a variety of subtle ways even if we are trying to mask it. They may not understand why there is tension in the relationship but they will probably feel it. Furthermore, frustration and tension impedes effective communication.

We can let go of our frustration when we recognize that patients aren't obligated to change in order to meet our needs. This recognition allows us to stop trying to persuade them to act the way we think they should and instead focus on helping them act the way they need in order to accomplish their goals.

About the Authors

Martha Mitchell Funnell, MS, RN, CDE, is a clinical nurse specialist and diabetes educator at the University of Michigan Diabetes Research and Training Center. She has won a number of honors and awards for her work in the areas of patient empowerment, patient education, and curriculum development. She is the American Diabetes Association's 2002–2003 President, Health Care & Education.

Robert M. Anderson, EdD, is an educational psychologist with 22 years of experience in diabetes research and education. He is an NIH-funded research scientist with the Michigan Diabetes Research and Training Center and professor of medical education at the University of Michigan Medical School. He has won a number of honors and awards for his work in diabetes education.

Nugget T. Burkhart, RN, MA, CPNP, CDE, is a practitioner in the Department of Pediatric Endocrinology at the University of Michigan. She coordinates the University of Michigan "Pump Team," a program for children and adolescents on insulin pump therapy. She works closely with children and their families to tailor their diabetes regimen to their specific and ever-changing needs.

Mary Lou Gillard, MS, RN, CDE, is a community nurse educator in the Department of Medical Education at the University of Michigan. She provides Diabetes Self-Management Education in a research setting and is the nurse case manager to those who participate in her program. She has had diabetes for 35 years.

Robin B. Nwankwo, MPH, RD, CDE, is a community dietitian employed by the Department of Medical Education at the University of Michigan. She coordinates grant-funded community complications screening and education programs.

About the American Diabetes Association

The American Diabetes Association is the nation's leading voluntary health organization supporting diabetes research, information, and advocacy. Its mission is to prevent and cure diabetes and to improve the lives of all people affected by diabetes. The American Diabetes Association is the leading publisher of comprehensive diabetes information. Its huge library of practical and authoritative books for people with diabetes covers every aspect of self-care—cooking and nutrition, fitness, weight control, medications, complications, emotional issues, and general self-care.

To order American Diabetes Association books: Call 1-800-232-6733. http://store.diabetes.org [Note: there is no need to use **www** when typing this particular Web address]

To join the American Diabetes Association: Call 1-800-806-7801. www.diabetes.org/membership

For more information about diabetes or ADA programs and services: Call 1-800-342-2383. E-mail: Customerservice@diabetes.org www.diabetes.org

To locate an ADA/NCQA Recognized Provider of quality diabetes care in your area: www.ncqa.org/dprp

To find an ADA Recognized Education Program in your area: Call 1-888-232-0822. www.diabetes.org/recognition/education.asp

To join the fight to increase funding for diabetes research, end discrimination, and improve insurance coverage: Call 1-800-342-2383. www.diabetes.org/advocacy

To find out how you can get involved with the programs in your community: Call 1-800-342-2383. See below for program Web addresses.

- *American Diabetes Month:* Educational activities aimed at those diagnosed with diabetes—month of November. www.diabetes.org/ADM
- *American Diabetes Alert:* Annual public awareness campaign to find the undiagnosed—held the fourth Tuesday in March. www.diabetes.org/alert
- *The Diabetes Assistance & Resources Program (DAR):* diabetes awareness program targeted to the Latino community. www.diabetes.org/ DAR
- *African American Program:* diabetes awareness program targeted to the African American community. www.diabetes.org/africanamerican
- *Awakening the Spirit: Pathways to Diabetes Prevention & Control:* diabetes awareness program targeted to the Native American community. www. diabetes.org/awakening

To find out about an important research project regarding type 2 diabetes: www.diabetes.org/ada/research.asp

To obtain information on making a planned gift or charitable bequest: Call 1-888-700-7029. www.diabetes.org/ada/plan.asp

To make a donation or memorial contribution: Call 1-800-342-2383. www.diabetes.org/ada/cont.asp